Sexual Function and Pelvic Floor Dysfunction

Angie Rantell

Editor

Sexual Function and Pelvic Floor Dysfunction

A Guide for Nurses and Allied Health Professionals

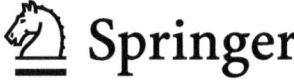 Springer

Editor
Angie Rantell
Urogynaecology Department
King's College Hospital
London
UK

ISBN 978-3-030-63842-9   ISBN 978-3-030-63843-6   (eBook)
https://doi.org/10.1007/978-3-030-63843-6

This Springer imprint is published by the registered company Springer Nature Switzerland AG
The registered company address is: Gewerbestrasse 11, 6330 Cham, Switzerland

Contents

Introduction

Angie Rantell

Sexual health is defined by the World Health Organisation (2006) as the integration of somatic, emotional, intellectual and social aspects in ways that are positively enriching and that will enhance personality, communication and love (World Health Organisation 2006). According to Masters and Johnson (1966), sexual function (SF) is defined as how the body reacts in different stages of the sexual response cycle. Sexual activity (SA) is the manner in which we express our sexuality. Optimal female sexual health comprises physical, mental and emotional aspects, and there are several variables that influence SF including physiological and psychosocial factors (Tsai et al. 2011).

Early research looking at female sexuality was conducted by Kinsey in 1953 (Kinsey 1953). The sexual practices of American men and women were studied to try to dispel the misconception that women are not interested in sex. It has been suggested that research on female sexuality lags behind research into male sexual function as some cultures have difficulty accepting that female sexual problems are as disruptive to a women's health-related quality of life (HRQL) as they are to a man's (Kingsberg and Althof 2009).

Widely held beliefs and assumptions about the aetiology of male sexual difficulties changed dramatically with the approval of Viagra (Sildenafil) in 1998, the first oral therapy for erectile dysfunction. Alongside enhancing the sexual performance of millions of men, the medical research its launch produced was equally dramatic. Today there is widespread acknowledgement of the multifaceted nature of sexual difficulties. For women, there has been no revolutionary medical treatment but interest and research into female sexual response, and sexual difficulties have grown steadily over the past two decades.

Pelvic floor dysfunction (PFD) is a term applied to a wide variety of clinical conditions, including urinary incontinence (UI), sensory and emptying

A. Rantell (✉)
Urogynaecology Department, King's College Hospital, London, UK
e-mail: angela.rantell@nhs.net

© Springer Nature Switzerland AG 2021   1
A. Rantell (ed.), *Sexual Function and Pelvic Floor Dysfunction*,
https://doi.org/10.1007/978-3-030-63843-6_1

abnormalities of the lower urinary tract, pelvic organ prolapse (POP), defecatory dysfunction, anal incontinence and several chronic pain syndromes (Bump and Norton 1998). Women may experience only one symptom or a combination of symptoms. The prevalence of women reporting at least one symptom of PFD is reported between 23.7 and 49.7% (Nygaard et al. 2008). The most common conditions are UI and POP. Urinary incontinence is thought to affect up to 70% of women at some point in their life (Milsom and Gyhagen 2019), and 50% of women will develop a pelvic organ prolapse (POP) in their lifetime (Smith et al. 2010). The prevalence for both of these problems increases with age and represents a significant problem for healthcare as the population ages. All of these individual conditions can have significant negative effects on women's quality of life and in particular they can significantly affect a woman's SF.

The prevalence of sexual dysfunction is estimated to be around 30–50% in the general population, whereas in women with PFD, the reported incidence rises to 50–83% (Verbeek and Hayward 2019). For women seeking help for PFD, it is essential to include a discussion and if appropriate an assessment of SF as part of a holistic assessment and treatment plan.

Nurses and Allied Health Professionals (AHPs) are key members of the multidisciplinary team providing care for women with PFD and are often ideally placed to not only initiate discussions with women regarding SF but also to offer support and advice. However, a lack of undergraduate and postgraduate training regarding sexual health and SF is a common problem for all healthcare professionals (HCPs), and this can negatively impact on the service that we can provide for our patients.

This book has been developed for nurses and AHPs with an interest in the care of women with PFD, but is relevant to all HCPs working with women. It is acknowledged that there are many different clinical conditions associated with PFD, and these are often compounded by common general gynaecological conditions, e.g. endometriosis, fibroids, gynaecological cancers. However, this book will focus solely on the most common pelvic floor conditions covering UI/lower urinary tract symptoms (LUTS) (including urinary tract infections (UTI), POP and genitourinary syndrome of menopause). It will not cover the anorectal aspects of PFD.

The two main aims of this book are:

1. To provide an overview of the most common conditions, reviewing the assessment, diagnosis and management of those conditions and understanding the impact that each of those conditions can have on SF.
2. To develop/enhance knowledge and skills related to SF history taking/assessment and holistic treatments.

The book is split loosely into five sections. Chapters 2 and 3 provide a background to SF, reviewing the physiology of SF and models of SF along with looking at definitions, terminology, prevalence and causes of sexual dysfunction.

Chapters 4–7 introduce four specific pelvic floor conditions. They will outline the condition, prevalence, causes, diagnosis and management of the individual conditions and provide a special focus on the impact of each individual condition on a woman's SF.

Chapters 8–10 aim to provide a guide on how to discuss SF with women, what a sexual assessment entails including history taking and physical examinations and finally will discuss the objective and subject measures available to enhance assessment and measure treatment success.

Chapters 11–14 will provide an overview of treatments available to holistically manage sexual dysfunction. The chapters will consider over the counter and home remedies, psychological therapies, physical therapies and pharmacological and surgical management options. For many, these chapters may provide a background to other therapies available and for some it may provide useful hints or guides to the evidence for particular therapies.

Finally, Chaps. 15 and 16 will consider the impact of partner issues on a woman's SF, and review help-seeking behaviours and signposting for specialist services that may be available for women to seek additional help.

It is hoped that by educating and demystifying the topic amongst HCPs, it will help to improve the recognition of problems in clinical practice and build HCP's confidence in initiating discussions regarding SF and providing ongoing care for women with PFD.

References

Bump RC, Norton PA (1998) Epidemiology and natural history of pelvic floor dysfunction. Obstet Gynecol Clin N Am 25(4):723–746

Kingsberg S, Althof S (2009) Evaluation and treatment of female sexual disorders. Int Urogynaecol J 20(suppl 1):S33–S43

Kinsey A (1953) Sexual behaviour in the human female. Saunders, Philadelphia

Masters W, Johnson V (1966) Human sexual response. Little Brown, Boston

Milsom I, Gyhagen M (2019) The prevalence of urinary incontinence. Climacteric 22(3):217–222

Nygaard I, Barber MD, Burgio KL, Kenton K, Meikle S, Schaffer J, Spino C, Whitehead WE, Wu J, Brody DJ, Pelvic Floor Disorders Network (2008) Prevalence of symptomatic pelvic floor disorders in US women. JAMA 300(11):1311–1316

Smith FJ, Holman CAJ, Moorin RE, Tsokos N (2010) Lifetime risk of undergoing surgery for pelvic organ prolapse. Obstet Gynecol 116(5):1096–1100

Tsai TF, Yeh CH, Hwang TI (2011) Female sexual dysfunction: physiology, epidemiology, classification, evaluation and treatment. Urol Sci 22(1):7–13

Verbeek M, Hayward L (2019) Pelvic floor dysfunction and its effect on quality of sexual life. Sex Med Rev 7(4):559–564

World Health Organisation (2006) Defining sexual health report of a technical consultation on sexual health. WHO, Geneva

Models of Sexual Response

2

Angie Rantell

2.1 Introduction

In order to understand sexual function in women, it is useful to consider the physiology of sexual function and the sexual response cycle. This chapter aims to discuss the sexual response models that have been developed over the years and consider the physiology of sexual response in women. It will also discuss how and why these have been refined over the years in line with advancing research, knowledge and understanding of female sexual function.

2.2 Early Sexual Response Models

The pioneering work of Dr. William Masters and Dr. Virginia Johnson in the 1960s expanded our knowledge and understanding of human sexual response. In laboratory conditions, they observed, monitored and assessed individuals and couples engaging in sexual activity and the research they produced formed the basis of a linear model of human sexual response that is still widely accepted today (Masters and Johnson 1966). This model identified four distinct phases and described the physiological changes that occurred in each phase. They believed that sexual problems occurred during breaks in this sexual response cycle and designed a treatment approach called 'sensate focus' therapy (Masters and Johnson 1970). In general, problems with sexual function were believed to be psychological or relational in origin. There were no variations considered for male and female response.

As shown in Fig. 2.1, the four phases described are excitement, plateau, orgasm and resolution. Sexual response will vary between different women and for an individual woman on different occasions. Women may not always reach the orgasmic

A. Rantell (✉)
Urogynaecology Department, King's College Hospital, London, UK
e-mail: angela.rantell@nhs.net

© Springer Nature Switzerland AG 2021
A. Rantell (ed.), *Sexual Function and Pelvic Floor Dysfunction*,
https://doi.org/10.1007/978-3-030-63843-6_2

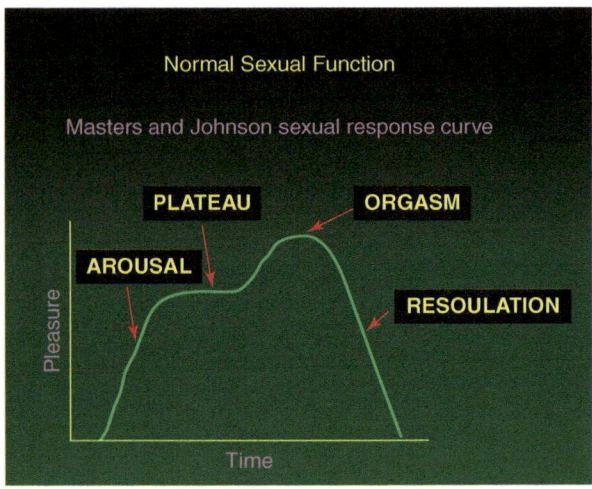

stage, and the resolution or refractory period is not always observed in women. If they do not experience a refractory period, women cannot respond to additional stimulation. However, in most cases women can respond to repeated stimulation and reach a second or third orgasm soon after the first (Chen et al. 2013).

Similar linear models by Kaplan (1979) and Leif (1977) were also introduced which added desire into the model; however, all these suggested that sexual response is invariant, the same for men and women, and that desire always precedes arousal.

2.3   Physiological Changes in the Sexual Response Cycle

The two basic physiological reactions that occur during sexual response are vaso-constriction of the genitalia and increased neuromuscular tension throughout the body (Masters and Johnson 1966). There are, however, a number of other physiological changes that happen to the female body as a result of sexual response, and these are described in Fig. 2.2 [adapted from Chen et al. 2013].

The desire phase is modulated by a balance of the dopamine-sensitive excitatory centre and the serotonin-sensitive inhibitory centre in the brain (Basson 2001). The activation of these centres initiates the downstream signals through the spinal cord and the related reflex centres producing a genital sexual response.

The parasympathetic nervous system mediates the engorgement of vascular and genital changes during the arousal phase. This includes the enlargement of the clitoris, dilation of perivaginal arterioles and expansion of the inner two-thirds of the vaginal canal (this is known as the tenting effect). At this point, transudation across the vaginal mucosa results in vaginal lubrication and this is regulated by oestrogen (Tsui et al. 2011).

The arousal phase is continued into the plateau phase. Plateau refers to the level of sexual excitement, which has been reached and is maintained for some time before reaching the orgasmic phase (Chen et al. 2013). This phase is associated with

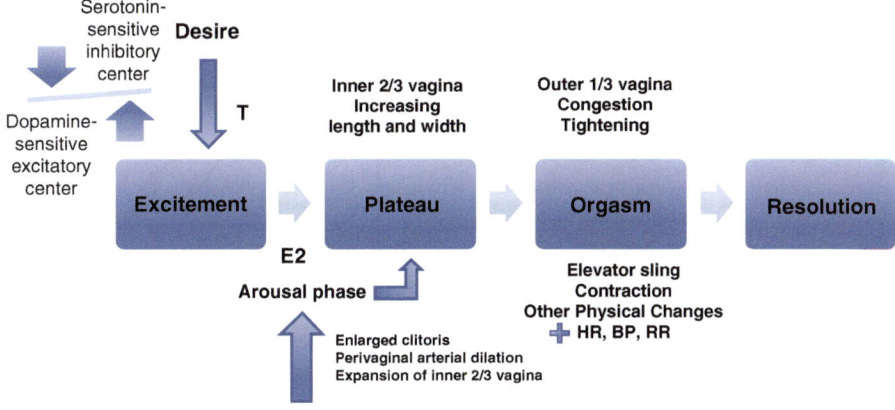

Fig. 2.2 Physiological changes in the current model of the female sexual response cycle (*BP* blood pressure, *HR* heart rate, *RR* respiratory rate). (With permission from Taiwanese Journal of Obstetrics and Gynecology)

expansion in the length and width of the inner two-thirds of the vagina, whilst the outer one-third of the vagina becomes congested with blood tightening the area. Masters and Johnson (1962) suggested that the congestion and tightening of the vagina was a feature of an orgasmic platform.

The orgasmic stage is not only associated with a series of contractions of the genital muscle groups (elevator sling/pelvic floor muscles) but also a general increase in neuromuscular tension throughout the body. This is also associated with an increase in heart rate, blood pressure and respiratory rate. Finally, during the refractory phase, the body returns to the unexcited state.

2.4   Further Development of Sexual Response Models

The early models described have been questioned over the years because they presume that men and women have similar sexual responses and do not take into account non-biological experiences such as pleasure and satisfaction or place sexuality in the context of a relationship (Whipple 2002; Whipple and Brash-McGregor 1997; Working Group on A New View of Women's Sexual Problems 2000). It is also noted that many women do not move progressively and sequentially through the phases as described. For example they may move from arousal to orgasm and satisfaction without experiencing sexual desire, or may experience desire, arousal and even satisfaction but not orgasm (Whipple 2002).

In 1997, Whipple and Brash-McGregor developed a circular sexual response model to address these issues (See Fig. 2.3 from Association of Reproductive Health Professionals (ARHP) 2008) (Whipple 2002; Working Group on A New View of Women's Sexual Problems 2000). This concept was built on four stages: seduction (encompassing desire), sensations (excitement and plateau), surrender (orgasm) and

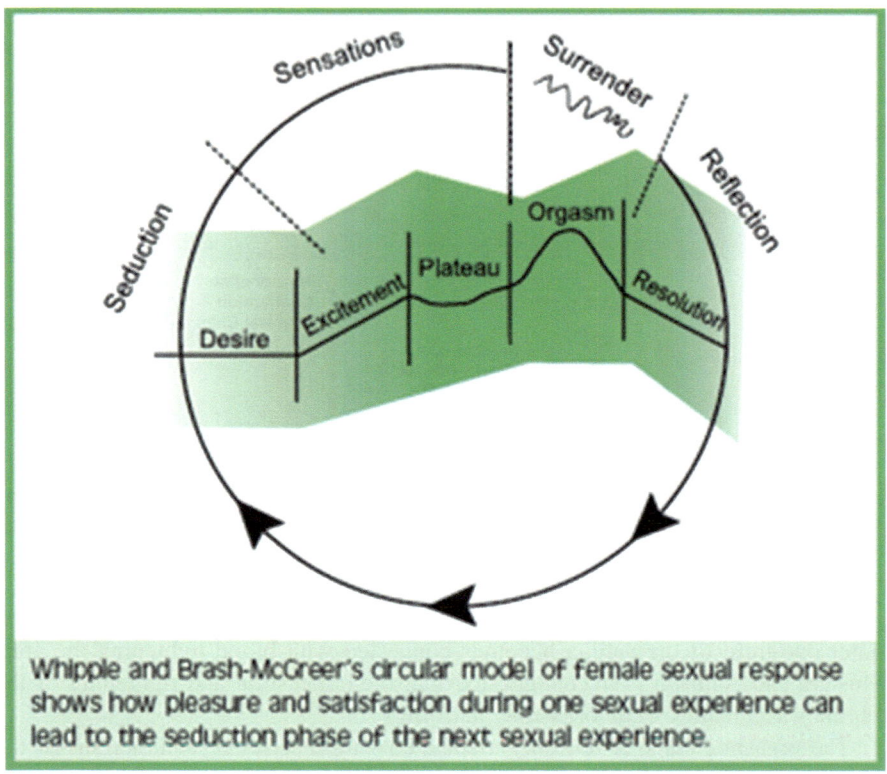

Whipple and Brash-McGreer's circular model of female sexual response shows how pleasure and satisfaction during one sexual experience can lead to the seduction phase of the next sexual experience.

Fig. 2.3 Circular model of female sexual response (ARHP 2008). (Developed by Whipple and Brash-McGregor 1997)

reflection (resolution). By making the model circular, it demonstrated that pleasant and satisfying sexual experiences may have a reinforcing effect on a woman, leading in to the seduction phase of her next sexual experience.

In 2000, Rosemary Basson revisited Masters and Johnsons linear model of human sexual response and argued that it did not adequately reflect the range of women's sexual responses and experience which she described as more complex and better described as a circular model of response affected by biological, psychological and relationship factors (ARHP 2008).

The model was refined into a non-linear model of female sexual response that incorporates the importance of emotional intimacy, sexual stimuli and relationship satisfaction and acknowledges that female functioning is significantly affected by psychosocial issues, e.g. satisfaction with the relationship, self-image and previous negative sexual experiences (Fig. 2.4) (ARHP 2008). It suggests that women begin a sexual encounter from a point of sexual neutrality and the decision to be sexually active comes from a conscious wish for emotional

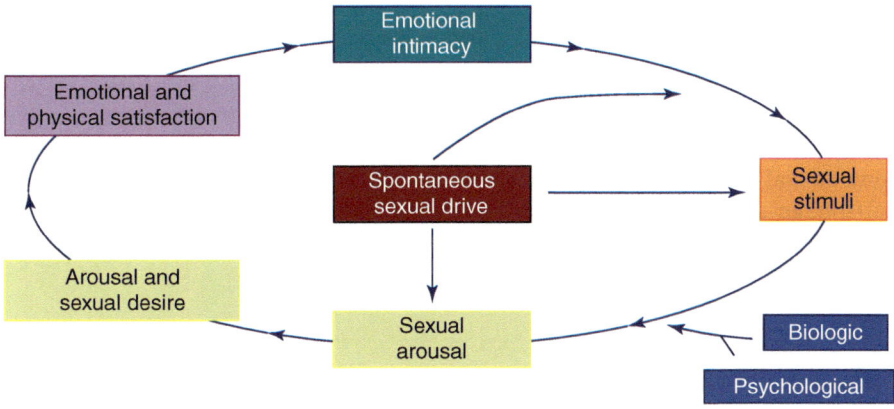

Fig. 2.4 Non-linear model of female sexual response (ARHP 2008)

closeness or as a result of seduction or suggestions from a partner (Kingsberg and Althof 2009). The empowering concept of this model is that of 'responsive desire' which suggests that the starting point for many women is one of neutrality or willingness to engage sexually as opposed to one of spontaneous desire. When a woman is open, responsive to touch and emotionally/physically connected to a partner, she begins to experience pleasure and 'responsive desire' (Metz et al. 2018). Ultimately, this model encompasses overlapping phases in a variable sequence and may be influenced by various psychological and physical factors during the process.

This remains the model most commonly used in current practice, and there are several key points that should be considered as noted below.

2.5   Key Points from Basson's Model

- 'Spontaneous sexual desire' is common in younger women and in the early months or years of a relationship but becomes more variable in the longer term.
- Women's subjective arousal is complex, often only minimally influenced by genital feedback and motivation to be sexual often stems from intimacy needs.
- Multiple biological factors can impact on a women's sexual response and inhibit sexual desire/interest and arousal.
- Desire/interest/arousal can be 'triggered' and is often contextual; resulting in the term 'responsive desire' commonly being used to help women understand that it is normal for some not to experience spontaneous sexual desire and help reframe the changes that can occur as a relationship progresses, as we age or in response to illness, medication or surgery.
- Desire/interest/arousal is often contextual, so how you experience sensation is context dependant and your perception can change depending on the context.

2.6 Sexual Desire/Motivation

Studies by Cain et al. (2003), Regan and Berscheid (1996) and Galyer et al. (1999) have revealed common motivations for women to agree to or initiate sex including a desire to: enjoy the emotional closeness that accompanies and follows sexual activity with a partner, increase their own sense of well-being and self-image and reduce guilt or anxiety about sexual infrequency. The importance of sex to a woman and man is also a considerable factor in female desire (DeLamater and Sill 2005).

2.7 Conclusions

Over the decades, it has been accepted that female sexual response is different to male sexual response, and models have been adapted to account for these differences. However, there are still many biological, psychological and contextual factors that can impact upon a woman's sexual function and many of these will be discussed later within this book. It is important to consider that many of these models may not be suitable or fit for all women, also how a woman moves through the models may vary for each woman throughout her life course.

Acknowledgement The author would like to acknowledge and Thank Angela Gregory for her contributions to the early sexual response models section and description and key points of Basson's model in this chapter.

References

ARHP (2008) Female sexual response – clinical fact sheet, Washington. http://www.arhp.org/Publications-and-Resources/Clinical-Fact-Sheets/Female-Sexual-Response

Basson RJ (2000) The female sexual response: a different model. J Sex Marital Ther 26:51–65

Basson R (2001) Female sexual response: the role of drugs in the management of sexual dysfunction. Obstet Gynaecol 98:350–353

Cain VS, Johannes CB, Avis NE (2003) Sexual functioning and practices in a multi-ethnic study of mid life women: baseline results from SWAN. J Sex Res 40:266–227

Chen CH, Lin YC, Chiu LH, Chu YH, Ruan FF, Liu WM, Wang PH (2013) Female sexual dysfunction: definition, classification, and debates. Taiwan J Obstet Gynecol 52(1):3–7

DeLamater JD, Sill M (2005) Sexual desire in later life. J Sex Res 42(2):138–149

Galyer KT, Conaglen HM, Hare A (1999) The effect of gyhnaecological surgery on sexual desire. J Sex Marital Ther 25:81–88

Kaplan H (1979) Disorders of sexual desire and other new concepts and techniques in sex therapy. Brunner Mazel, New York

Kingsberg S, Althof S (2009) Evaluation and treatment of female sexual disorders. Int Urogynaecol J 20(suppl 1):S33–S43

Leif H (1977) Inhibited sexual desire. Med Aspectsw Hum Sex 7:94–95

Masters WH, Johnson VE (1962) The sexual response cycle of the human female. III. The clitoris: anatomic and clinical consideration. West J Surg Obstet Gynecol 70:248–257

Masters WH, Johnson VE (1966) Human sexual response. Churchill, London

Masters WH, Johnson VE (1970) Human sexual inadequacy. Churchill, London

Metz M, Epstein N, McCarthy B (2018) Cognitive-behavioural therapy for sexual dysfunction. Taylor & Francis, New York

Regan P, Berscheid E (1996) Belief about the state, goals and objects of sexual desire. J Sex Marital Ther 22:110–120

Tsui KH, Wang PH, Chen CK, Chen YJ, Chiou SH, Sung YJ et al (2011) Non-classical estrogen receptors action on human fibroblasts. Taiwan J Obstet Gynecol 50:474–478

Whipple B (2002) Women's sexual pleasure and satisfaction. A new view of female sexual function. Female Patient 27:39–44

Whipple B, Brash-McGregor K (1997) Management of female sexual dysfunction. In: Sipski ML, Alexander CJ (eds) Sexual function in people with disability and chronic illness. A health professional's guide. Aspen Publishers, Gaithersbyrg, pp 509–534

Working Group on A New View of Women's Sexual Problems (2000) Electronic J Hum Sex 3. https://doi.org/www.ejhs.org

What Is Female Sexual Dysfunction?

3

Angie Rantell

3.1 Definitions/Classifications of Female Sexual Dysfunction (FSD)

The American Diagnostic and Statistical Manual of Mental Disorders (DSM) is the most frequently used and widely adopted diagnostic criteria for sexual disorders. In the first two versions of the DSM in 1952 and 1968, the concept of FSD did not exist and only the terms frigidity and vaginismus were included in a list of supplementary terms (Graham 2016). As medicine was a very male dominated field at that time, it could be suggested that it was not considered important or that women had not felt able to raise their concerns due to societal/gender constraints. At this time, little had changed since the famous Imlach case of the nineteenth century, where the woman sued a gynaecologist for loss of sexual function after her ovaries were removed and the male dominated jury had to decide if the ovaries were important (Morantz-Sanchez 2000). It took a further 20–30 years to break down these barriers for FSD to be defined and classified, and many of these new classifications were led by women.

According to the WHO International Classifications of Diseases-10 (ICD-10), the definition of FSD includes 'the various ways in which an individual is unable to participate in a sexual relationship as she would wish' (World Health Organisation (ICD-10) 1992). FSD can afflict women of any age and its expression changes with the endocrinology of advancing years (Buster 2013).

In 1998, The Sexual Function Health Council of the American Foundation for Urological Disease (AFUD) compiled the first consensus-based definition and classification system for FSD. They listed five major categories of dysfunction: desire, aversion, arousal, orgasmic and sexual pain disorders (Basson et al. 2000). These are further defined in Table 3.1 (Aslan and Fynes 2008).

A. Rantell (✉)
Urogynaecology Department, King's College Hospital, London, UK
e-mail: angela.rantell@nhs.net

© Springer Nature Switzerland AG 2021
A. Rantell (ed.), *Sexual Function and Pelvic Floor Dysfunction*,
https://doi.org/10.1007/978-3-030-63843-6_3

Table 3.1 Categories of dysfunction

Sexual disorders	Definition
Hypoactive sexual desire disorder	The persistent or recurrent deficiency of sexual fantasies/thoughts and/or receptivity to sexual activity that causes personal distress
Sexual aversion disorder	The persistent or recurrent phobic aversion to and avoidance of sexual contact with a sexual partner that causes personal distress
Sexual arousal disorder	The persistent or recurrent inability to attain or maintain sufficient sexual excitement causing personal distress
Orgasmic disorder	The persistent or recurrent difficulty, delay in or absence of attaining orgasm after sufficient sexual stimulation and arousal which causes personal distress
Sexual pain disorders	Recurrent or persistent genital pain associated with sexual intercourse, including dyspareunia, vaginismus and non-coital pain disorders

Fig. 3.1 The vicious cycle of FSD

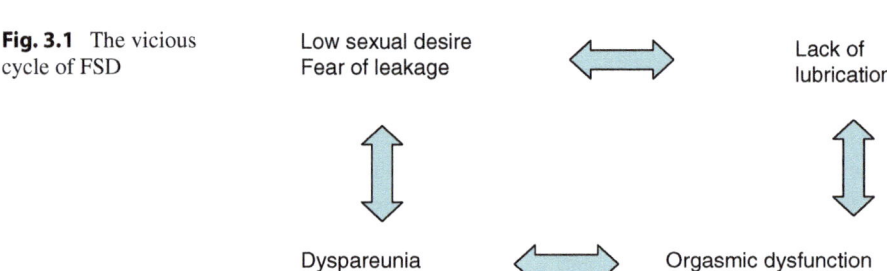

These classifications, which may coexist, are subtyped as life-long versus acquired, generalised versus situational and organic versus psychogenic (Basson et al. 2000). FSD is not always a primary pathology but may be a symptom or a side effect of another, for example pelvic floor dysfunction (Basson et al. 2005). Mouritsen (2009) reported on the 'vicious cycle' of FSD and how all areas may be interlinked (see Fig. 3.1).

Following on from this, the DSM-IV defined FSD as 'disturbances in sexual desire and in the psychophysiological changes that characterise the sexual response cycle and cause marked distress and interpersonal difficulty' (American Psychiatric Association 2000).

The classification of FSD was further updated in 2004 at the Second International Consensus of Sexual Medicine, and guidelines were established to aid clinicians to evaluate the clinical significance of symptoms and further define the distress (Basson 2005).

However, throughout the literature, many comments have been made regarding difficulties defining FSD in practice and when a sexual problem should be classified as a sexual dysfunction (Bancroft et al. 2003; Chen et al. 2013; Latif and Diamond 2013). Bancroft and Graham (2011) suggest that the specific challenge is the recognition of the marked variability of women's sexual experiences and the need to distinguish between transient problems in SF, e.g. due to adaptive responses to stressful circumstances and more persistent problems. Over a 10-year period, a task force and working group for the American Psychiatric Association (APA) updated diagnostic categories and criteria for FSD. The DSM-IV was revised and the DSM-V (2013) was adopted. Within this update, the definition of sexual dysfunctions was changed to 'a group of disorders that are typically characterised by a clinically significant disturbance in a person's ability to respond sexually or to experience sexual pleasure' (American Psychiatric Association 2013). Their symptoms should have been present for at least 6 months and been experienced in 75–100% of sexual encounters. The classification of female sexual desire disorder was removed, and female arousal disorder was re-named female interest/arousal disorder to cover a more varied expression of sexual desires in females. Sexual aversion disorder was also removed due to rare use and lack of supporting evidence. Changes to terminology were also introduced and dyspareunia was revised to genital pelvic pain, and the classification of vaginismus was replaced with the term penetration disorder (Chen et al. 2013; Derogatis et al. 2010). As with all terminology changes, they have been made to make terms more generalisable (e.g. genital pelvic pain), more specific (e.g. penetration disorder) or to come in line with new evidence. There are pros and cons to each of these in terms of broadening or narrowing diagnosis for patients; however, this can only make a difference if clinicians are educated about the new terminology and advised about how this may change outcomes for patients or the treatments offered to them. Yet, in current practice in the UK, these terms are not well known and not used in routine clinical practice.

3.2   Prevalence of FSD

Difficulties estimating the prevalence of FSD in women have been reported, and this is thought to be due to the fact that the parameters of FSD are not as clear as those of male sexual dysfunction (MSD) (Laumann et al. 1999) and because it is hard to determine the level of distress associated with sexual symptoms in a large-scale survey (Nappi et al. 2016). Methods of evaluating FSD and outcomes assessments have varied widely between studies (Hayes et al. 2006) and it has been suggested that many place an overemphasis on genital response rather than a subjective assessment of arousal and desire (Graham 2010) or even whether the event was sexually satisfying despite a limited genital response. Prevalence data suggest that the rates of FSD in clinical populations (i.e. women attending gynaecology clinics) are between 40 and 50% (Laumann et al. 1999; Geiss et al. 2003; Nazareth et al. 2003). However, there are very few studies looking at the prevalence of FSD in 'real world' populations, probably due to the difficulties accessing this population and the intimate nature of the subject being investigated. Ventegodt (Ventegodt 1998) performed an anonymised assessment of QoL amongst 2460 representative Danish women, which included five SF questions (out of a total of 317 questions). They found that the QoL of individuals with sexual problems was between 1.2 and 19.1% lower than the population means (range of population mean QoL 61.5–75.9, range of women with sexual problems mean QoL 57.3–67.5). Lack of sexual desire and lack of a suitable partner were the two most commonly cited sexual problems for women; however, no data were provided relating the sexual problems to age of the respondent, relationship satisfaction and general health to be able to further comment or justify the reduced QOL.

The Global Study of Sexual Attitudes and Behaviour included 27,500 women over the age of 40 from 29 countries and considered the prevalence of FSD according to geographical location. It was reported that lack of interest in sex varied from 17% in Europe to 34% in Southeast Asia, lubrication problems ranged from 12% in Europe and the Middle East to 28% in Asia. Pain during intercourse ranged from 5% in Europe to 22% in Southeast Asia and the inability to reach orgasm varied from 10% in Europe to 34% in Southeast Asia (McCabe et al. 2016). This study suggests that women in Southeast Asia report the most sexual problems. This could potentially be for a variety of reasons, for example the respondents in these surveys may not have been representative of the population especially given the rural nature of this part of the world or possibly issues with how the questions were translated. Laumann et al. (2005) reported early ejaculation and erectile dysfunction to be more prevalent amongst men from Southeast Asia than other parts of the world and that 20% of men in Southeast Asia lacked interest in sex. This may also have a significant impact of the sexual health of the women in the region. It is also important to consider the cultural and socio-economic aspects that may contribute to these high figures as there is a significant prostitution/sex trafficking issue in that area that may also be impacting upon women's long-term sexual function.

Ponholzer et al. (2005) studied the prevalence and risk factors for FSD in a cohort of women undergoing a voluntary health assessment as part of a public health initiative. A total 703 women between the ages of 20 and 80 years completed a questionnaire on FSD; 22% reported desire disorders, 35% arousal disorders and 39% orgasmic problems, all of these issues increased significantly with age and 12.9% reported pain disorders but this was more common amongst the 20–39 age group. However, this study still relied on women volunteering to participate and disclose sensitive information and is unlikely to represent the population.

Wolpe et al. (2017) performed a systematic review to assess the prevalence of FSD in Brazil. They reported that the prevalence of FSD ranged from 13.3 to 79.3% of the population studied. When considering the specific aspects of FSD, they found that sexual desire concerns ranged from 11 to 75%, arousal from 8 to 68.2%, lubrication from 29.1 to 41.4%, orgasm from 18 to 55.4% and satisfaction from 3.3 to 42%. It was suggested that the range in prevalence occurred due to the differences in the populations studied, for example age, marital status, educational level, family income and associated comorbidities.

3.3   Causes of FSD

Gladu (2002) reported four causes of FSD: medical illnesses, psychological ill-nesses, hormonal deficiencies or the effects of medications. Examples of these causes can be found in Table 3.2. Sociocultural and relationship-related causes have also been linked with dissatisfaction or discontent with sexual experiences (Tiefer et al. 2002). It is likely that in many cases, no one single factor will be the cause but a combination of multiple factors.

Buster (2013) developed a table of all the medications associated with FSD which was adapted from the ARHP (2005). As demonstrated, many groups of drugs have the potential to impact upon SF, and Table 3.3 displays which drugs have the potential to cause desire, arousal or orgasmic disorders.

Mouritsen (2009) also suggested areas of pathophysiology that can cause FSD (Fig. 3.2).

Low oestrogen levels in the vagina, urethra, trigone epithelium and atrophy of the pelvic floor muscles have also been proposed as causes for FSD and lower uri-nary tract symptoms (LUTS) (Bligic and Beji 2010). Oral contraceptives have been shown to reduce arousal and sexual interest and increase genito-pelvic pain in women (Lee et al. 2017).

Several studies have reported increased FSD in women with higher body mass index (BMI) (Assimakopoulos et al. 2006; Esposito et al. 2007; Bond et al. 2009). A recent study by Mostafa et al. (2018) reported that in young, premenopausal population, obese women were more likely to have desire, arousal and lubrication problems compared to overweight women. However, the discussion did not con-sider whether this was due to hormonal/medical causes or psychological causes, e.g. reduced body image/low self-esteem or functional issues with sexual activity due to body habitus.

Nazarpour et al. (2016) performed a systematic review to identify factors affect-ing SF following menopause. Table 3.4 demonstrates some of the factors identified. Although, this study only assessed women during the menopause, it highlights the complexity of the physical, emotional, social and interpersonal and intrapersonal factors that can all impact upon FSD. These factors represent significant challenges in all research in SF as it is impossible to exclude all the compounding variables.

Table 3.2 Causes of FSD in women

Medical illnesses	Psychological illnesses	Hormonal deficiencies	Effects of medications
Hypertension Diabetes Thyroid dysfunction Neurological demyelinating conditions Previous pelvic surgery	Depression Anxiety Bipolar disorders Schizophrenia	Menopausal changes Female androgen deficiency syndrome	Selective serotonin reuptake inhibitors Antidepressants Antihypertensives Tamoxifen Phenothiazines

Table 3.3 Medications associated with FSD

Medication	Desire disorder	Arousal disorders	Orgasm disorders
Psychotropics			
Antipsychotics	+		+
Barbiturates	+	+	+
Benzodiazepines	+	+	
Lithium	+	+	+
SSRIs	+	+	+
TCA	+	+	+
MAO inhibitors			+
Trazodone	+		
Venlafaxine	+		
Cardiovascular and antihypertensive medications			
Antilipid medications	+		
Beta blockers	+		
Clonidine	+	+	
Digoxin	+		+
Spironolactone	+		
Methyldopa	+		
Hormonal preparations			
Danazol	+		
GnRH agonists	+		
Hormonal contraceptives	+		
Antiandrogens	+	+	+
Tamoxifen	+	+	
GnRH analogues	+	+	
Ultralight contraceptive pills	+	+	
Other			
Histamine H2 receptor blockers	+		
Indomethacin	+		
Ketoconazole	+		
Phenytoin sodium	+		
Aromatase inhibitors	+	+	
Chemotherapeutic agents	+	+	
Anticholinergics		+	
Antihistamines		+	
Amphetamines and related anorexic drugs			+
Narcotics			+

SSRIs selective serotonin reuptake inhibitors, *TCA* tricyclic antidepressants, *MAO* monoamine oxidase inhibitors

Fig. 3.2 Areas of
pathophysiology of sexual
dysfunction

Areas of pathophysiology of sexual dysfunction

- Mind and age (neurotransmitters, medication)
- Vaginal epithelium and lubrication
- Vaginal blood flow
- Coital incontinence
- Scar tissue / vaginal dimensions
- Neuropathy
- Pelvic floor muscles

Table 3.4 Factors affecting SF

Physical factors	Psychological/emotional/social factors	Relationship/partner factors
Age	Depression	Partners' sex problems
Oestrogen deficiency	Anxiety	Quality of relationship with
Type of menopause	Smoking	spouse
Chronic medical problems	Alcohol	Partners' loyalty
Severity of menopausal	Access to healthcare	Sexual knowledge
symptoms	Poor understanding of women's	History of divorce or
Dystocia history	health	widowhood
Health status		Living apart from spouse

3.4   Psychosocial Factors

It has been observed that there is a significant interaction between communication and sexual satisfaction (Litzinger and Gordon 2005; Mota 2017; Montesi et al. 2013; McNulty et al. 2016) and that these interpersonal factors play a major role in maintenance of sexual problems (Derogatis et al. 2010), yet marital satisfaction and communication with partners was not addressed in this study. Pascoal et al. (2014) performed an exploratory study to understand how lay people define sexual satisfaction and identified two themes. The first was in relation to sexual pleasure including arousal, orgasm and sexual openness, the second theme emphasised relational dimensions including romance, expression of feelings and mutuality and that both areas are crucial to sexual satisfaction.

Schoenfeld et al. (2017) also reported that husbands' positive interpersonal behaviour towards their wives improved sexual satisfaction. According to Rehman et al. (2013), women tend to be more sexually satisfied, if they are older, in a stable long-term relationship, are more erotophilic (respond to sexual cues in a positive manner) and have better sexual and non-sexual communication with their partner.

3.5 Controversies in the Diagnosis of FSD in Women with Pelvic Floor Dysfunction

A variety of studies have demonstrated the prevalence and impact of FSD in women with pelvic floor disorders. However, with the update of the DMS-V in 2013, not only was the terminology and classification changed but new criteria for the diagnosis of FSD were added (Graham 2016). Female sexual dysfunction now includes the following criterion: 'the sexual dysfunction is not better explained by a nonsexual mental disorder or as a consequence of severe relationship distress or other significant stressors and it is not attributable to the effects of a substance/medication or another medical condition' (APA 2013: 424). Given this criterion, sexual disturbances associated with incontinence or any other pelvic floor disorder should not be classified as a sexual dysfunction, even if they cause personal suffering and distress (Mota 2017).

For many women, sexual difficulties may be multifactorial, and the presence of pelvic floor dysfunction may not be bothersome or impact on their sexual functioning so it raises the question of how to differentiate which factors impact the most on sexual functioning, in order to define a dysfunction or disorder?

3.6 Conclusions

SF is a complex process that includes physical, social and emotional factors. FSD appears to be a prevalent condition in clinical populations; however, the true prevalence in the general population is still not known. It can, however, have a significant impact on a woman's QoL and relationships. The challenges in assessing the prevalence of FSD in the general population include language variations, cultural differences and access to all populations. As there are so many variables, it may only be possible to research certain groups of women individually. Given that research into this field has only started to develop over the past 40 years, it could also be considered that the definitions are still dominated by a 'male' model of sexual functioning rather than fully recognising the underlying psychological and emotional factors that are essential to a woman's SF.

References

American Psychiatric Association (2000) Diagnostic and statistical manual of mental disorders – text revision fourth ed (DSM-IV-TR). American Psychiatric Association, Washington, DC

American Psychiatric Association (2013) Diagnostic and statistical manual of mental disorders (DSM-5®). American Psychiatric Publication, Philadelphia

Aslan E, Fynes M (2008) Female sexual dysfunction. Int Urogynaecol J 19:293–305

Assimakopoulos K, Panayiotopoulos S, Iconomou G, Karaivazoglou K, Matzaroglou C, Vagenas K, Kalfarentzos F (2006) Assessing sexual function in obese women preparing for bariatric surgery. Obes Surg 16(8):1087–1091

Association of Reproductive Health Professionals (ARHP) (2005) Women's sexual health in midlife and beyond. Clin Pract 5:8–12

Bancroft J, Graham CA (2011) The varied nature of women's sexuality: unresolved issues and a theoretical approach. Horm Behav 59(5):717–729

Bancroft J, Loftus J, Long J (2003) Distress about sex: a national survey of women in heterosexual relationships. Arch Sex Behav 32:193–204

Basson R (2005) Women's sexual dysfunction: revised and expanded definitions. Can Med Assoc J 172(10):1327–1333

Basson R, Berman J, Burnett A, Derogatis L, Ferguson D, Fourcroy J, Goldstein I, Garziottin A, Heiman J et al (2000) Report of the International Consensus development conference on female sexual dysfunction. J Urol 163(3):888–893

Basson R, Brotto LA, Laan E, Redmond G, Utian WH (2005) Women's sexual dysfunctions: assessment and management of women's sexual dysfunctions: problematic desire and arousal. J Sex Med 2(3):291–300

Bligic D, Beji N (2010) Lower urinary tract symptoms in women and quality of life. Int J Urol Nurs 4(3):97–105

Bond DS, Vithiananthan S, Leahey TM, Thomas JG, Sax HC, Pohl D, Ryder BA, Roye GD, Giovanni J, Wing RR (2009) Prevalence and degree of sexual dysfunction in a sample of women seeking bariatric surgery. Surg Obes Relat Dis 5(6):698–704

Buster JE (2013) Managing female sexual dysfunction. Fertil Steril 100(4):905–915

Chen CH, Lin YC, Chiu LH, Chu YH, Ruan FF, Liu WM, Wang PH (2013) Female sexual dysfunction: definition, classification, and debates. Taiwan J Obstet Gynecol 52(1):3–7

Derogatis LR, Laan E, Brauer M, Van Lunsen RH, Jannini EA, Davis SR, Fabre L, Smith LC, Basson R, Guay AT, Rubio-Aurioles E (2010) Responses to the proposed DSM-V changes. J Sex Med 7(6):1998–2014

Esposito K, Ciotola M, Giugliano F, Bisogni C, Schisano B, Autorino R, Cobellis L, De Sio M, Colacurci N, Giugliano D (2007) Association of body weight with sexual function in women. Int J Impot Res 19(4):353–357

Geiss I, Umek W, Dungl A (2003) Prevalence of female sexual dysfunction in gynaecologic and urogynaecologic patients according to the International Consensus Classification. Urology 62:514–518

Gladu R (2002) Female sexual dysfunction: classification, physiology, diagnosis and treatment. J Sex Reprod Med 2(1):21–27

Graham CA (2010) The DSM diagnostic criteria for female sexual arousal disorder. Arch Sex Behav 39(2):240–255

Graham CA (2016) Reconceptualising women's sexual desire and arousal in DSM-5. Psychol Sex 7(1):34–47

Hayes RD, Bennett CM, Fairley CK, Dennerstein L (2006) Epidemiology: what can prevalence studies tell us about female sexual difficulty and dysfunction? J Sex Med 3(4):589–595

Latif EZ, Diamond MP (2013) Arriving at the diagnosis of female sexual dysfunction. Fertil Steril 100(4):898–904

Laumann E, Palk A, Rosen R (1999) Sexual dysfunction in the United States. JAMA 281(6):537–544

Laumann EO, Nicolosi A, Glasser DB, Paik A, Gingell C, Moreira E, Wang T (2005) Sexual problems among women and men aged 40–80 y: prevalence and correlates identified in the Global Study of Sexual Attitudes and Behaviors. Int J Impot Res 17(1):39

Lee JJM, Low LL, Ang SB (2017) Oral contraception and female sexual dysfunction in reproductive women. Sex Med Rev 5(1):31–44

Litzinger S, Gordon KC (2005) Exploring relationships among communication, sexual satisfaction, and marital satisfaction. J Sex Marital Ther 31(5):409–424

McCabe MP, Sharlip ID, Lewis R, Atalla E, Balon R, Fisher AD, Laumann E, Lee SW, Segraves RT (2016) Incidence and prevalence of sexual dysfunction in women and men: a consensus statement from the Fourth International Consultation on Sexual Medicine 2015. J Sex Med 13(2):144–152

McNulty JK, Wenner CA, Fisher TD (2016) Longitudinal associations among relationship satisfaction, sexual satisfaction, and frequency of sex in early marriage. Arch Sex Behav 45(1):85–97

Montesi JL, Conner BT, Gordon EA, Fauber RL, Kim KH, Heimberg RG (2013) On the relationship among social anxiety, intimacy, sexual communication, and sexual satisfaction in young couples. Arch Sex Behav 42(1):81–91

Morantz-Sanchez RM (2000) Conduct unbecoming a woman: medicine on trial in turn-of-the-century Brooklyn. Oxford University Press on Demand, New York

Mostafa AM, Khamis Y, Helmy HK, Arafa AE, Abbas AM (2018) Prevalence and patterns of female sexual dysfunction among overweight and obese premenopausal women in Upper Egypt; a cross sectional study. Middle East Fertil Soc J. 23(1):68–71

Mota RL (2017) Female urinary incontinence and sexuality. Int Braz J Urol. 43(1):20–28

Mouritsen L (2009) Pathophysiology of sexual dysfunction as related to pelvic floor disorders. Int Urogyneacol J 20(suppl 1):S19–S25

Nappi RE, Cucinella L, Martella S, Rossi M, Tiranini L, Martini E (2016) Female sexual dysfunction (FSD): prevalence and impact on quality of life (QoL). Maturitas 94:87–91

Nazareth I, Boynton P, King M (2003) Problems with sexual function in people attending London general practitioners: cross sectional study. BMJ 23:327–423

Nazarpour S, Simbar M, Tehrani FR (2016) Factors affecting sexual function in menopause: a review article. Taiwan J Obstet Gynecol 55(4):480–487

Pascoal PM, Narciso IDSB, Pereira NM (2014) What is sexual satisfaction? Thematic analysis of lay people's definitions. J Sex Res 51(1):22–30

Ponholzer A, Rochlich M, Racz U, Temml C, Madersbacher S (2005) Female sexual dysfunction in a healthy Austrian cohort: prevalence and risk factors. Eur Urol 47:366–375

Rehman US, Fallis E, Byers ES (2013) Sexual satisfaction in heterosexual women. An essential handbook of women's sexuality. ABC-CLIO vol 1, pp 25–45

Schoenfeld EA, Loving TJ, Pope MT, Huston TL, Štulhofer A (2017) Does sex really matter? Examining the connections between spouses' nonsexual behaviors, sexual frequency, sexual satisfaction, and marital satisfaction. Arch Sex Behav 46(2):489–501

Tiefer L, Hall M, Tavris C (2002) Beyond dysfunction: a new view of women's sexual problems. J Sex Marit Ther 28(S1):225–232

Ventegodt S (1998) Sex and the quality of life in Denmark. Arch Sex Behav 27(3):295–307

Wolpe RE, Zomkowski K, Silva FP, Queiroz APA, Sperandio FF (2017) Prevalence of female sexual dysfunction in Brazil: a systematic review. Eur J Obstet Gynecol Reprod Biol 211:26–32

World Health Organisation (ICD-10) (1992) International statistical classification of diseases and related health problems. WHO, Geneva

Impact of Incontinence on Female Sexual Function

4

Victoria Kershaw and Swati Jha

4.1   Background

Women suffering from urinary symptoms, and incontinence in particular, have a high prevalence of sexual dysfunction. Female reproductive and urinary systems share anatomical structures and neurovascular innervation, and disorders of both often share aetiology, thus urological and sexual problems commonly coexist. Arguably more significant however is the impact that urinary symptoms such as incontinence can have on female body image which in turn negatively influences sexuality. In this chapter, we will learn more about common conditions affecting the lower urinary tract and explore their impact on quality of life, psychological health and sexual function.

Lower urinary tract symptoms (LUTS) are extremely common. The lower urinary tract refers to the bladder and urethra whereas the upper urinary tract encompasses the kidneys and ureters. One large international population study found that in women aged ≥40, 76.3% had at least one LUTS 'sometimes' and 52.5% had at least one LUTS 'often' (Coyne et al. 2009). Regarding incontinence specifically, a UK population-based study showed a total of 40% of respondents suffered urinary incontinence, which caused significant problems in 8.5% (Cooper et al. 2014).

Lower urinary tract symptoms can be divided into three categories:

- Storage symptoms: e.g. frequency, urgency, dysuria, nocturia, stress incontinence, urge incontinence.

Author Contributions:
VK: Researched and wrote the chapter, editing and approval of final version
SJ: Senior author on chapter, researched and wrote the chapter, editing and approval of final version

V. Kershaw · S. Jha (✉)
Sheffield Teaching Hospitals NHS Foundation Trust, Sheffield, UK
e-mail: Swati.Jha1@nhs.uk

© Springer Nature Switzerland AG 2021   23
A. Rantell (ed.), *Sexual Function and Pelvic Floor Dysfunction*,
https://doi.org/10.1007/978-3-030-63843-6_4

- Voiding symptoms: e.g. poor stream, hesitancy, terminal dribbling, overflow incontinence (due to chronic urinary retention).
- Postmicturition symptoms: e.g. incomplete emptying, postmicturition dribble.

Women complain of more storage symptoms than voiding symptoms, whereas men are more likely to have voiding symptoms (Robinson et al. 2012).

Some of the LUTS women may experience are:

- Dysuria: Burning or other discomfort during micturition. Discomfort may be intrinsic to the lower urinary tract or external (vulvar dysuria).
- Bladder pain: Suprapubic or retropubic pain, pressure or discomfort, related to the bladder, and usually increasing with bladder filling. It may persist or be relieved by voiding.
- Frequency: Micturition occurs more frequently during waking hours than previously deemed normal by the woman.
- Urgency: A sudden, compelling desire to pass urine which is difficult to defer.
- Incontinence: Involuntary loss of urine.
- Nocturia: Interruption of sleep one or more times because of the need to urinate. Each void is preceded and followed by sleep, i.e. not awake for another reason.
- Hesitancy: Delay in initiating micturition.
- Slow stream: Urinary stream perceived as slower than previous performance or in comparison to others.
- Straining to void: The need to make an intensive effort (by abdominal straining, Valsalva or suprapubic pressure) to initiate, maintain or improve the urinary stream.
- Incomplete emptying: The bladder does not feel empty after micturition.
- Postmicturition dribbling: A further involuntary passage of urine following the completion of micturition.
- Urinary retention: The inability to pass urine despite persistent effort.
- Polyuria: Overproduction of urine, associated with diabetes mellitus, diabetes insipidus, chronic kidney disease.
- Nocturnal polyuria: Excess proportion of urine excretion occurring during the night (over 20–30% of total 24 h voided volume, age dependent).
- Haematuria: Blood in urine (which can be visible or non-visible).

N.B. These definitions are in line with the International Urogynecological Association (IUGA)/International Continence Society (ICS) Joint Report on the Terminology for Female Pelvic Floor Dysfunction 2010 (Haylen et al. 2010).

4.2　Causes of Lower Urinary Tract Symptoms

There are several possible causes of LUTS; however, in many cases no specific cause is found.

Cause	Mechanism	Lower urinary tract symptoms
Urinary tract infection (UTI)	Bacterial infection of the bladder (cystitis)	Dysuria, frequency, urgency, urgency urinary incontinence, bladder pain, cloudy/smelly urine and haematuria
Genital prolapse	Distortion of pelvic anatomy Although surgical repair does not guarantee improvement in LUTS	Frequency, urgency stress incontinence, incomplete bladder emptying and recurrent UTIs Stress incontinence may occur for the first time after prolapse repair 'occult incontinence'
Genitourinary syndrome of the menopause (GSM)	Hypoestrogenism of urothelium leading to thinning and inflammation as seen in vulvovaginal atrophy	Frequency, urgency, dysuria and recurrent UTIs
Pelvic mass, e.g. fibroid uterus, ovarian tumour	Pressure on the lower urinary tract	Frequency, urgency and stress urinary incontinence
Bladder stones (calculi)	May irritate bladder mucosa and potentially obstruct flow of urine	Bladder pain, dysuria, frequency, nocturia, haematuria and difficulty passing urine
Bladder malignancy	Tumour bleeds into urine Bladder mucosa becomes irritated and inflamed Location of tumour may potentially obstruct flow of urine	Haematuria (visible or non-visible) is the most common presentation Frequency, urgency, nocturia and dysuria Difficulty passing urine, urinary retention
Bladder pain syndrome/interstitial cystitis	Disruption of the bladder mucosa surface layer and damage of its glycosaminoglycan (GAG) component, exposing subepithelial layer to urinary toxins, resulting in neurogenic inflammation and chronic bladder epithelial damage (Arslan et al. 2019)	Bladder pain particularly related to bladder filling, urgency and frequency
Medication side effects: Anticholinergics, e.g. tricyclic antidepressants, antihistamines, opiates Alpha blockers, antipsychotics Diuretics, lithium, caffeine, alcohol	Inhibit detrusor contraction Relaxation of bladder neck Increase urinary production by the kidney	Urinary retention ± overflow incontinence Urinary incontinence, particularly stress incontinence Frequency, urgency, urgency incontinence

4.2.1 Urinary Incontinence

Urinary incontinence is broadly categorised into three groups: urgency urinary incontinence (UUI), stress urinary incontinence (SUI) and mixed urinary incontinence (MUI). Risk factors for urinary incontinence include age, genitourinary syndrome of the menopause, obesity, number of children, prolonged labour, heavy lifting, genital prolapse, chronic cough, constipation, family history of incontinence and radiotherapy.

4.2.1.1 Overactive Bladder

Overactive bladder (OAB) is a syndrome consisting of a combination of symptoms including urinary urgency, with or without urgency incontinence, usually with urinary frequency and nocturia, in the absence of UTI or other obvious pathology. OAB is subdivided into OAB wet (i.e. with urgency incontinence) and OAB dry (i.e. urgency but no incontinence). The overall prevalence of OAB is reported to be 16.6% and increases with advancing age (Jha et al. 2012). When this is caused by an involuntary bladder contraction seen on a urodynamics test, then it is known as detrusor overactivity (DO). Symptoms may occur unpredictably but there may also be reproduceable triggers such as putting the key in the door arriving home, or turning on taps and listening to running water.

Bladder training and lifestyle modifications are the first-line of treatment. Lifestyle modifications may include: avoidance of caffeine, alcohol and foods that may irritate the bladder (e.g. citrus and tomatoes), smoking cessation (bladder irritant), fluid intake modification and weight loss if needed. Medication may also be prescribed. Pharmacological and surgical management of OAB is discussed further in Chap. 14.

The majority of DO cases are idiopathic; however, neurological conditions such as multiple sclerosis (MS) and spinal cord injury (SCI) can be associated with a severe 'neurogenic' form. In these specific patients, increased bladder storage pressure can put the upper urinary tract at risk of deterioration, and reducing this risk is a primary aim of therapy. Urinary incontinence is reported by approximately 50% of MS patients, 52.3% with SCI, 33.1% with Parkinson's disease and 23.6% with stroke (Castagna et al. 2015). A neurological examination is essential if there is any suspicion that LUTS may be due to an underlying neurological condition.

4.2.1.2 Stress Urinary Incontinence

Stress urinary incontinence (SUI) is the most common form of incontinence. It is defined by IUGA/ICS as the involuntary loss of urine on effort or physical exertion, or on sneezing or coughing (Haylen et al. 2010). Urinary leakage occurs in the presence of an increase of intra-abdominal pressure in the absence of micturition desire. It is caused by either a deficiency in the function of the urinary sphincter itself or/ and weakness in the pelvic floor musculature that supports the urethra and bladder, leading to urethral hypermobility. When these mechanisms fail and with an increase of intra-abdominal pressure (such as laughing, weight lifting, cough, sneezing), incontinence occurs. Pregnancy and parturition are the most common causes of pelvic floor muscle weakness and resultant SUI. However, any mechanism of chronically increased intra-abdominal pressure can also lead to pelvic floor weakness including chronic constipation, chronic cough and obesity.

The first-line treatment for stress incontinence is supervised pelvic floor exercises and weight loss if needed. If this fails, the patient may be offered surgical management, which is discussed further in Chap. 14.

4.2.1.3 Mixed Urinary Incontinence

Patients with mixed urinary incontinence (MUI) suffer from both overactive bladder symptoms and stress urinary incontinence. In MUI, one of the incontinence types is often more bothersome than the other. This is referred to as urgency predominant MUI or stress predominant MUI depending on which symptom is most problematic. These patients are likely to need to undergo treatment for both conditions. Bladder training, OAB medication and pelvic floor physiotherapy can all be undertaken simultaneously. Before undergoing surgery for stress urinary incontinence, it is best practice to first control any symptoms of OAB as it is possible that this may be exacerbated by SUI surgery.

4.2.1.4 Other Causes of Urinary Incontinence

Overflow incontinence occurs as a result of chronic urinary retention. When the bladder becomes full, it leaks a small amount of urine 'overflow' without prior warning. The patient will also have signs and symptoms of voiding dysfunction and urinary retention in addition to incontinence, e.g. a feeling of incomplete bladder emptying or a persistent desire to void.

If a patient reports continuous urinary leakage without urgency or an increase in intra-abdominal pressure, it is important to consider the possibility of a vesicovaginal fistula (an abnormal connection between the bladder and vagina in which urine drains from the bladder into the vagina and out of the body). This is a rare condition that may occur following gynaecological surgery, gynaecological cancer, radiotherapy or obstructed labour in developing countries.

Nocturnal enuresis is involuntary loss of urine that occurs only during sleep at night. It is more common in children than adults.

In this overview of LUTS, we have outlined a range of symptoms and causes. It is important to highlight at this point that LUTS not only have implications for the physical health of women but also carry a significant psychological, social and economic burden. This is discussed in more depth later in the chapter.

4.3   Investigation of Lower Urinary Tract Symptoms

- *Physical examination:* is guided by the history and may include abdominal palpation, vaginal examination and potentially neurological assessment.

- *Quality of life (QOL) questionnaires:* may be used to quantify the severity of symptoms and impact they are having on the patient's life. They include Bristol Female Lower Urinary Tract Symptoms (BFLUTS), Incontinence Quality of Life (I-QoL), Electronic Personal Assessment Questionnaire Pelvic Floor (ePAQ-PF) and King's Health Questionnaire (KHQ).
- *Urinalysis:* signs of infection include leucocytes, nitrates and potentially protein and blood. It is important to ensure there is no glycosuria as undiagnosed diabetes may potentially be an underlying cause of LUTS. Persistent microscopic haematuria can be a sign of bladder cancer.
- *Urine Microscopy, Culture and Sensitivity (MC + S):* if urinalysis detects signs of a UTI, the sample may be sent for MC + S. If a particular bacteria is cultured, this can then help to guide antibiotic therapy for the patient.
- *Postvoid residual:* this is when a bladder scan is used to measure the volume of urine remaining in the bladder after the patient has voided. It is used to ensure the patient is fully emptying their bladder. A normal value is <50 ml, though some consider <100 ml to be more acceptable.
- *3-day bladder diary:* also known has a frequency/volume chart. The patient is asked to measure and record their fluid intake, urinary output, episodes of incontinence and symptoms of urgency over 3 days. This can help to quantify frequency, nocturia and severity of incontinence, as well as identify targets for modification such as timing and volume of fluid intake.
- *Ultrasound urinary tract:* may be indicated to rule out underlying problems in the upper urinary tract such as ureteric obstruction or resultant renal cortical scarring in a patient with recurrent UTIs.
- *Cystoscopy:* cystoscopy is performed when it is necessary to rule out bladder malignancy or calculi, for example in the case of haematuria, recurrent UTIs or refractory OAB. The majority of patients can tolerate the procedure comfortably under local anaesthetic. If a suspicious lesion is seen, a biopsy is performed and sent for histological examination.
- *Urodynamics:* is a test designed to examine bladder pressures during filling, provocation and emptying. X-rays may also be performed during the test (videourodynamics). A dual lumen catheter is placed in the bladder to facilitate both bladder filling and also measurement of vesical pressure. A second catheter is placed in either the rectum or the vagina to measure abdominal pressure. A graphical record of vesical pressure, abdominal pressure and detrusor pressure (vesical—abdominal) is produced. In the provocation phase, attempts are made to recreate the patient's symptoms, for example coughing to demonstrate stress incontinence or turning on the taps to trigger urgency. Detrusor overactivity is diagnosed if there is an involuntary rise in detrusor pressure which may be spontaneous or provoked. Urodynamic stress incontinence is diagnosed when there is involuntary leakage of urine with increased intra-abdominal pressure in the absence of a detrusor contraction.

4.4   Impact of Urinary Incontinence on Quality of Life

Urinary symptoms may exact a heavy toll on quality of life. Incontinence is a particularly embarrassing and potentially disabling condition which may affect social, psychological, occupational, domestic, physical and sexual aspects of life. In severe cases, urinary incontinence may lead to complete social isolation, depression and decline in general health.

Due to its largely unpredictable nature, OAB tends to have larger repercussions regarding quality of life measures; however, severe stress incontinence which occurs with minimal exertion and/or in large volumes has the potential also to drastically reduce a person's ability to work, travel, sleep, exercise, socialise and participate in intimate relationships. Women with MUI report lower quality of life scores than women with either isolated OAB or SUI and tend to be the most severely affected group.

The impact that urinary incontinence can have on quality of life may also negatively influence mental health. Women with all types of urinary incontinence show lower mental health scores, but MUI is associated with the lowest scores (poorest mental health). Women report higher degrees of low mood, sadness and loneliness compared to the general healthy population. Urinary incontinence is associated with anxiety, depression and dissatisfaction with life. The depression rate in patients with urinary incontinence is comparable to patients with chronic illnesses such as diabetes and heart disease. The psychological effects of urinary incontinence appear to be more severe in younger patients (Mallah et al. 2014).

The effect of urinary incontinence on the quality of life of women can vary according to religious beliefs. For example, urinary incontinence can have a more devastating effect on Muslim women as it breaches women's status of ritual 'purity' (Mallah et al. 2014).

There is also a significant economic burden to women, not only in potential restrictions to working life but also in the cost of pad usage and frequent changing and washing of clothing.

4.5   Urinary Incontinence and Sexual Function

There is considerable evidence demonstrating the impact of urinary incontinence on sexual function, the fact that urinary and sexual symptoms are often comorbid, and that attention to urinary problems may enhance sexual quality of life. All women with lower urinary tract symptoms are at increased risk of sexual dysfunction, and the odds of sexual dysfunction increase as the urinary symptoms become more complex and severe (Chen et al. 2013).

4.5.1 Prevalence of Female Sexual Dysfunction

The majority of women consider sexuality to be a fairly or very important matter in their life. However, half of women suffering from incontinence stated that their sexual life was spoiled to some degree by their urinary problems (Nilsson et al. 2011). Prevalence of FSD in women with incontinence is reported to be 46–68% depending on the source. This is compared to the background prevalence of female sexual dysfunction, which is reported between 30 and 60% in various studies. Indeed, 5% of women with incontinence avoid intercourse altogether (Visser et al. 2014).

Interestingly in a study of Swedish couples in which the women suffer from urinary incontinence or OAB, 50% of the women reported that urinary symptoms had a negative impact on their sex lives whereas only 20% of their partners did, suggesting there is some discrepancy in the perception of the impact on sexual function between the sexes (Nilsson et al. 2011).

4.5.2 Impact of Urinary Incontinence on Sexual Function

Common sexual complaints in women with incontinence include decreased sexual desire, lubrication problems, anorgasmia and dyspareunia (Zahariou et al. 2010). This was categorised further according to DSM-IV criteria by Salonia et al. in 2004, who reported that in a cohort of incontinent women 34% reported hypoactive sexual desire, 23% reported sexual arousal disorder, 11% reported orgasmic disorder and 44% reported sexual pain disorder (Salonia et al. 2004).

Vaginal dryness and lack of lubrication can be caused by the presence of urine in the vagina which affects normal acidic pH as well as urine dermatitis of the vulva.

Concerns regarding malodour, needing to dispose of pads prior to intercourse and fear of urinary leakage during coitus can lead to reduced self-esteem, altered body image and feelings of being less attractive to their partner (Zahariou et al. 2010).This may in turn result in a lower frequency of sexual activity, avoidance of sex or experiencing less pleasure and freedom during sex (Jha et al. 2012; Zahariou et al. 2010). Women expressed that they require more time for arousal and also to achieve orgasm because of an inability to relax. These problems are highly personal issues and women often feel ashamed of their symptoms and are unlikely to share their concerns with their partner. Ultimately the ramifications of urinary incontinence can negatively impact relationships with partners and for women without partners, their confidence to find a partner. Unfortunately, urinary symptoms may eventually lead to cessation of sexual activity for some women (Castagna et al. 2015). Younger sexually active women with incontinence have the most to lose, and they tend to complain of greater sexual distress than their older counterparts.

In a study examining the impact on sexual function for patients with urodynamic proven incontinence, those who leaked during urodynamic studies had worse sexual function than those who did not. It is likely that patients who leak during urodynamics have worse urinary incontinence than those who are unable to reproduce their physiological symptoms during the test, suggesting that worse urinary symptoms correlate with worse sexual function (Cohen et al. 2008).

The symptom of nocturnal incontinence is independently associated with lack of sexual activity (Tannenbaum et al. 2006).

To avoid urinary leakage during intercourse, women may adopt methods that decrease sexual satisfaction, such as interrupting intercourse to void.

4.5.3   OAB Versus SUI

When considering the difference in sexual function between patients with OAB and SUI; studies are conflicting but on the whole, the effect of OAB is generally reported to be worse than the effect of SUI. Women with MUI report significantly worse sexual function, however, than those with either UUI or SUI, when matched for age, parity and BMI (Coksuer et al. 2011).

Women with OAB complain of repeated experiences of needing to void and having to interrupt sexual activity to go to the toilet. This is known as 'coital urinary urgency' according to IUGA/ICS definition (Rogers et al. 2018). Urgency incontinence causes distress and discomfort because urine leakage is unpredictable and unavoidable. Women with urgency incontinence often lose urine during orgasm, which according to patients is particularly upsetting. Incontinence may make some women feel unclean and, consequently, undesirable.

The EpiLUTS study showed that OAB with UUI (OAB-wet) was associated with a greater likelihood of decreased sexual activity and decreased sexual enjoyment than OAB without UUI (OAB-dry) (Coyne et al. 2011). In another study, patients with OAB-dry had more desire for sexual activity, better vaginal lubrication, achieved orgasm more frequently and reported higher sexual satisfaction scores than patients with OAB-wet, MUI or SUI (Coyne et al. 2009).

4.5.4   Coital Incontinence

Coital incontinence, i.e. loss of urine during or after vaginal intercourse, is surprisingly prevalent with up to 65% of women with urinary incontinence reporting this symptom (Zahariou et al. 2010).

Urinary incontinence related to coitus has been described in two ways: urinary leakage occurring on vaginal penetration and urinary leakage at the time of orgasm (Rogers et al. 2018). Penetration urinary incontinence is more strongly associated with SUI and is probably related to intrinsic urethral sphincter. Orgasmic urinary incontinence is more associated with overactive bladder, although there is overlap in both groups. Coital incontinence has been reported in up to 89% of women with SUI compared to 33% of women with OAB (Serati et al. 2009).

Although there is no consistent anatomical abnormality detected in women with coital incontinence, urodynamic studies performed during orgasm in healthy women have demonstrated involuntary bladder contractions and urethral relaxation. It is conceivable that these orgasm-related effects may predispose women with already tenuous continence mechanisms (urethral sphincter incompetence, OAB, etc.) to have coital incontinence (Chen et al. 2013).

4.5.5 Sexual Pain Disorder

Women with urinary incontinence report a high prevalence of sexual pain disorder. This seems to affect women with OAB and bladder pain syndrome in particular.

In a study by Zahariou, which examined the effect of OAB on sexual function, 47% of incontinent women indicated that they experienced bothersome pain in their abdominal/ genital area during intercourse. These results are consistent with other studies. The underlying cause of sexual pain in these patients has not been fully investigated. Urine dermatitis and lack of lubrication are likely to be contributory factors to dyspareunia. Anxiety regarding urinary incontinence or odour may also play a role in terms of pelvic floor spasm (Zahariou et al. 2010).

Patients with bladder pain syndrome report the highest sexual pain scores of all women with LUTS. Pelvic pain due to inflammation of the bladder wall and neuropathic dysfunction, dyspareunia and fear of pain during intercourse are particularly common amongst this group of people and may cause resistance to penetration and consequent pelvic floor overactivity, vulvodynia and vaginismus (Sacco et al. 2012).

4.5.6 Impact of Intercourse on Urinary Symptoms

As many as 40% of women cite sexual intercourse as an instigating or exacerbating event for urinary symptoms. This is known as 'post coital LUT symptoms' according to IUGA/ICS definition and may encompass worsening symptoms of urinary frequency or urgency, dysuria and suprapubic tenderness (Rogers et al. 2018). This is a particular problem for patients with recurrent UTIs who may suffer from post-coital UTIs specifically. Another group of note is patients who suffer from bladder pain syndrome, in which intercourse is a well-recognised trigger for symptoms. Indeed, the number of patients who choose to abstain from intercourse because of the effect on urinary symptoms is particularly high in those suffering from bladder pain syndrome (Chen et al. 2013).

4.6 Management of Sexual Function in Women with LUTS

This is discussed comprehensively in Chaps. 13 and 14. A few key points are highlighted below.

A dialogue about sexual function in women with urinary symptoms should become an integral component in clinical practice. Education and advice may yield sexual function benefits in nearly every setting. Timed voiding, education of the patient and her partner on the benignity of exposure to sterile urine, fluid avoidance and/or voiding immediately prior to sexual activity and use of sexual lubricants may help sexual function in virtually any type of urinary syndrome.

Conservative treatment of urinary incontinence using pelvic floor muscle training has been shown to present an improvement in the domains of desire, arousal and orgasm, regardless of the type of urinary incontinence. It has also been demonstrated to improve coital incontinence, particularly in patients with SUI.

Medical and surgical therapy for urinary issues may have a positive effect on sexual function by mitigating distressing symptoms. However, treatment-related side effects or complications may attenuate sexual function gains or even worsen sexual function overall. Careful patient counselling and documentation of baseline sexual function are required before any therapy for urinary symptoms.

4.7 Conclusions

Urinary incontinence, irrespective of the cause, plays an important part in sexual dysfunction and they often coexist. The management of UI may improve FSD, but cannot be guaranteed to do so and on occasion some of the surgical treatments for SUI have been found to cause de-novo FSD. Patients should be warned of this when proceeding with surgery, to ensure realistic expectations of outcomes. However, coital incontinence appears to be positively affected, and overall the treatment of UI has a positive impact on FSD.

Disclosure of Interests VK: none relevant to publication
SJ: none relevant to publication

References

Arslan B et al (2019) Outcomes of intravesical chondroitin-sulfate and combined hyaluronic-acid/chondroitin-sulfate therapy on female sexual function in bladder pain syndrome. Int Urogynecol J 30:1857–1862

Castagna G, Montorsi F, Salonia A (2015) Chapter 10 Sexual and bladder comorbidity in women. In: Handbook of clinical neurology, vol 130. Elsevier, Amsterdam, pp 165–176

Chen J, Sweet G, Shindel A (2013) Urinary disorders and female sexual function. Curr Urol Rep 14:298–308

Cohen BL, Barboglio P, Gousse A (2008) The impact of lower urinary tract symptoms and urinary incontinence on female sexual dysfunction using a validated instrument. J Sex Med 5:1418–1423

Coksuer H et al (2011) Does urinary incontinence subtypes affect sexual function? Eur J Obstet Gynecol Reprod Biol 159:213–217

Cooper J et al (2014) Prevalence of female urinary incontinence and its impact on quality of life in a cluster population in the United Kingdom (UK): a community survey. Prim Health Care Res Dev 16:377–382

Coyne KS et al (2009) The prevalence of lower urinary tract symptoms (LUTS) in the USA, the UK and Sweden: results from the Epidemiology of LUTS (EpiLUTS) study. BJU Int 104:352–360

Coyne KS et al (2011) The impact of OAB on sexual health in men and women: results from EpiLUTS. J Sex Med 8:1603–1615

Haylen BT et al (2010) An International Urogynecological Association (IUGA)/International Continence Society (ICS) joint report on the terminology for female pelvic floor dysfunction. Neurourol Urodyn 29:4–20

Jha S, Ammenbal M, Metwally M (2012) Impact of incontinence surgery on sexual function: a systematic review and meta-analysis. J Sex Med 9:34–43

Mallah F et al (2014) Effect of urinary incontinence on quality of life among Iranian women. J Fam Reprod Heal 8:13–19

Nilsson M, Lalos O, Lindkvist H, Lalos A (2011) How do urinary incontinence and urgency affect women's sexual life? Acta Obstet Gynecol Scan 90:621–628

Robinson D, Staskin D, Laterza RM, Koelbl H (2012) Defining female voiding dysfunction: ICI-RS 2011. Neurourol Urodyn 31:313–316

Rogers RG et al (2018) An International Urogynecological Association (IUGA)/International Continence Society (ICS) joint report on the terminology for the assessment of sexual health of women with pelvic floor dysfunction. Neurourol Urodyn 37:1220–1240

Sacco E et al (2012) Bladder pain syndrome associated with highest impact on sexual function among women with lower urinary tract symptoms. Int J Gynecol Obstet 117:168–172

Salonia A et al (2004) Sexual dysfunction is common in women with lower urinary tract symptoms and urinary incontinence: results of a cross-sectional study. Eur Urol 45:642–648

Serati M, Salvatore S, Uccella S, Nappi RE, Bolis P (2009) Female urinary incontinence during intercourse: a review on an understudied problem for women's sexuality. J Sex Med 6:40–48

Tannenbaum C, Corcos J, Assalian P (2006) The relationship between sexual activity and urinary incontinence in older women. J Am Geriatr Soc 54:1220–1224

Visser E, Bock GH, Berger MY, Dekker JH (2014) Impact of urinary incontinence on sexual functioning in community-dwelling older women. J Sex Med 11:1757–1765

Zahariou A, Karamouti M, Tyligada E, Papaioannou P (2010) Sexual function in women with overactive bladder. Female Pelvic Med Reconstr Surg 16:31–36

Impact of Pelvic Organ Prolapse on Sexual Function

5

Sushma Srikrishna and Angie Rantell

5.1 Introduction

Prolapse (Latin: Prolapsus—'a slipping forth') refers to a falling, slipping or downward displacement of a part or organ. Pelvic organ refers most commonly to the uterus and/or the different vaginal compartments and their neighbouring organs such as bladder, rectum or bowel. Pelvic organ prolapse (POP) is thus, primarily, a definition of anatomical change (Haylen et al. 2016). In other words, POP refers to the loss of support to the uterus, bladder and/or bowel leading to their descent from their normal anatomic position towards or through the vaginal introitus (Giarenis et al. 2014).

Urogenital prolapse is a common distressing condition with a significant adverse impact on quality of life (QoL) (Kelleher et al. 1997; Digesu et al. 2005). Large population studies suggest that the prevalence of stage 3–4 prolapse is in the range of 2–11% (Swift 2000; Swift et al. 2005a; Slieker-ten et al. 2004).

5.2 Aetiology of Pelvic Organ Prolapse

The aetiology of pelvic organ prolapse is multifactorial, resulting from loss of the support maintained by a complex interaction amongst the levator ani, the vagina and the connective tissue, as well as neurologic injury from stretching of the pudendal nerves that may occur during childbirth. The known and suspected risk factors implicated in the aetiopathogenesis of POP are summarised in the table below.

S. Srikrishna (✉)
King's College Hospital, London, UK
e-mail: sushmasrikrishna@nhs.net

A. Rantell
Urogynaecology Department, King's College Hospital, London, UK

© Springer Nature Switzerland AG 2021
A. Rantell (ed.), *Sexual Function and Pelvic Floor Dysfunction*,
https://doi.org/10.1007/978-3-030-63843-6_5

Vaginal delivery, advancing age and increasing body mass index are the most consistent risk factors.

Increasing vaginal parity has been demonstrated to be the strongest risk factor for pelvic organ prolapse in women younger than 60 years (Mant et al. 1997). The Women's Health Initiative (Hendrix et al. 2002) noted that single childbirth was associated with raised odds of uterine prolapse (odds ratio 2:1; 95% CI 1.7–2.7), cystocoele (2:2; 1.8–2.7) and rectocele (1:9; 1.7–2.2). Every additional delivery up to five births increased the risk of worsening prolapse by 10–20%. Similarly, the Pelvic Organ Support study has also shown the increased risk of POP with increasing parity (Swift et al. 2005b). Caesarean section seems to protect against prolapse development whereas forceps delivery enhances risk. A long-term national Swedish cohort study has shown that the prevalence of POP was doubled after vaginal delivery compared with caesarean section, two decades after one birth. Increasing infant birthweight and current BMI were also significant risk factors for POP after vaginal delivery (Gyhagen et al. 2013).

Both incidence and prevalence of pelvic organ prolapse increase with advancing age (Hunskaar et al. 2005). The relative prevalence of this disorder rises by about 40% with every decade of life (Hagen et al. 2004). Surgery for prolapse is uncommon in people younger than 30 and older than 80 years; for women between these ages, incidence rises steadily (Hagen et al. 2009; Olsen et al. 1997a).

Increasing body mass index is also implicated in the development of pelvic organ prolapse. Women who are overweight (BMI 25–30 kg/m^2) and obese (>30 kg/m^2) are at high risk of developing this disorder (Abrams et al. 2005; Moroni et al. 2019). Similarly, overweight women are more likely to undergo surgery for prolapse (Moalli et al. 2003).

Box 5.1 Established and Potential risk factors for POP

Established risk factors
Vaginal delivery
Advancing age
Obesity
Potential risk factors
Obstetric factors
Pregnancy (irrespective of mode of delivery)
Forceps delivery
Young age at first delivery
Prolonged second stage of labour
Infant birthweight >4500 g
Shape or orientation of bony pelvis
Family history of pelvic organ prolapse
Race or ethnic origin
Occupations entailing heavy lifting
Constipation
Connective-tissue disorders
Previous hysterectomy

5.3   Symptomatology of POP

Many women with objective prolapse are asymptomatic and do not need treatment. Conversely, symptom bother may be considerable in some women. The most common symptoms associated with POP are those of a vaginal lump or bulge, or a 'dragging' sensation. Equally, POP may present with secondary symptoms suggestive of bladder involvement or bowel impairment. POP can also cause sexual dysfunction, which is discussed in some detail in this chapter.

5.3.1   Summary Overview of Primary and Secondary Symptoms

Primary:
- Vaginal lump or bulge
- Dragging sensation

Secondary:
- Straining to void, intermittent stream (due to urethral compression or kinking)
- Straining at stool, incomplete bowel emptying and digitation
- Recurrent urinary tract infections (due to incomplete emptying resulting in a chronic residual volume)
- Nocturia (due to accumulating residuals during the day)

The commonest prolapse-specific sexual symptoms that lead women to seek medical help are summarised below in Table 5.1 (Rogers et al. 2018).

5.4   Sexual Dysfunction in POP

Women with advanced POP are more likely to feel self-conscious and less physically and sexually attractive than women without this condition (Jelovsek and Barber 2006). About one-third of sexually active women with POP report that their condition interferes with sexual function (Weber et al. 1995; Barber et al. 2002).

The prevalence of sexual dysfunction is estimated to be around 30–50% in the general population, whereas in women with pelvic floor dysfunction, the reported incidence rises to 50–83% (Verbeek and Hayward 2019). Sexual dysfunction is also

Table 5.1 Prolapse - specific sexual symptoms

Symptoms	Definition
Abstinence due to pelvic organ prolapse	Physical or psychological reason why a woman or her partner does not engage in sexual activity due to prolapse or associated symptoms
Obstructed intercourse	Vaginal intercourse that is difficult or not possible due to obstruction by genital prolapse or shortened vagina
Vaginal laxity	Feeling of vaginal looseness
Vaginal wind	Passage of air from the vagina (usually accompanied by sound)

common in women attending urogynaecology clinics, with up to 64% of sexually active women reporting dissatisfaction with their sex life (Pauls et al. 2006). Sexual function in this population of women has been shown to be adversely affected in a number of studies (Mant et al. 1997; Salonia et al. 2004; Handa et al. 2004; Lukacz et al. 2007), although data are limited and conflicting. Some studies suggest that women with coexistent lower urinary tract symptoms are significantly more likely than those without urinary symptoms to report decreased libido and dyspareunia (Gyhagen et al. 2013). In addition, possible confounding variables such as older age and postmenopausal status may alter the association between prolapse and sexual function (Dennerstein et al. 2003). Finally, a significant proportion of women with urogenital prolapse may not be sexually active and therefore sexual function in this group is very difficult to assess.

5.5   Pathophysiology of Sexual Dysfunction in Women with Urogenital Prolapse

A review of literature reveals conflicting views regarding the impact of urogenital prolapse on female sexual function. Several pathophysiological mechanisms have been proposed to explain female sexual dysfunction in association with urogenital prolapse. These include urogenital atrophy, obstruction caused by physical presence of the prolapse, a short or narrow vagina or a tense contracted pelvic floor. Lack of physical sexual response may lead to discomfort and pain, aggravated by lack of lubrication and genital swelling. Psychological factors such as lack of libido or negative emotional reactions associated with sex, embarrassment or fear of urinary or faecal leakage, leading to avoidance of sex could also play a part. Severe prolapse can be associated with urinary or faecal incontinence which in turn has an added negative impact on sexual function (Ellerkmann et al. 2001).

5.6   Physical Presence of Prolapse

The actual presence of an obstructive bulge in the vagina or a sense of vaginal laxity may itself lead to sexual dysfunction, particularly in more severe degrees of prolapse. During coitus, vaginal dimensions and compliance increase and decreased vaginal length, width or elasticity caused by prolapsed vaginal tissue, scarring from previous surgery or mesh insertion can cause dyspareunia. However, even patients with moderate prolapse may remain asymptomatic for sexual problems.

Some studies have shown a relationship between increasing degrees of prolapse and interference with sexual activity (Slieker-ten et al. 2004; Moalli et al. 2003; Handa et al. 2008), although not with sexual pleasure or frequency of sexual intercourse. Interestingly, although there is evidence to suggest a correlation between impairment of sexual function and worsening prolapse (Moalli et al. 2003), surgical correction may not necessarily improve sexual function (Helström and Nilsson 2005).

5.7   Associated Local Pathology

Long-standing prolapse may be associated with skin excoriation, keratinisation or even ulceration in severe cases. In association with urinary incontinence, there may be poor skin condition, particularly inflamed ammoniacal dermatitis. In additions, vaginal and urinary tract infections are quite common in postmenopausal women. All of these factors can be implicated in sexual dysfunction.

5.8   Genito-Urinary Syndrome of Menopause [GSM]

The urogenital organs, urethra, bladder, vagina and vulva, are highly oestrogen dependent, as is the blood flow to the pelvis. Therefore, vulvovaginal atrophy commonly occurs in the postmenopausal state, leading to a loss of the vaginal epithelial integrity and loss of normal vaginal microflora. This results in a thinning of the vaginal epithelium and bacterial overgrowth caused by the loss of the acidic state provided by the normal premenopausal flora. Loss of blood flow to the pelvic organs results in decreased vaginal lubrication during the normal sex response cycle, resulting in dyspareunia. In addition, there is an increased incidence of vaginal and urinary tract infections. Decreased lubrication problems and consequent dyspareunia is also related to the level of oestrogen. Systemic oestrogen therapy has been shown to improve libido, lubrication and orgasm in postmenopausal women (Berman et al. 1999; Sarrel et al. 1998). Local vaginal oestrogen has also been shown to significantly improve vaginal atrophy, dryness, lubrication and urinary urgency, which are commonly seen in conjunction with urogenital prolapse (Suckling et al. 2003).

Although there have been some reports which suggest that a reduced vaginal blood flow may contribute to sexual dysfunction, oestrogens have not been proven to increase vaginal blood flow (Laan et al. 2003). GSM is discussed in more detail in Chap. 7.

5.9   Psychological Factors

Evidence shows that body image is important to a woman's perceived quality of life. Her perception of her feelings of self-consciousness, femininity and physical and sexual attractiveness may be important emotional factors to consider in women suffering from advanced pelvic organ prolapse (Swift et al. 2005a). It is well known that the physiology of sexual function is very complex and is associated with multiple factors in addition to normal functional anatomy. Sexual desire and orgasmic capabilities have been shown to have an inverse relationship with anxiety states (Hartmann et al. 2004). Conversely, previous qualitative studies on urogenital prolapse have not detected significant psychological issues in women with prolapse, in sharp contrast to those caused by incontinence (Teunissen et al. 2006), apart from lack of confidence in some women, or a sense of 'being unattractive' or 'less womanly' in others. Other studies conclude that prolapse does not seem to interfere with genital body image or with sexual function (Moroni et al. 2019), hence data are conflicting.

5.10 Associated Incontinence

Women seldom volunteer symptoms of urinary leakage during intercourse. However, urogenital prolapse can frequently be associated with urinary incontinence, which has a significant impact on sexual dysfunction. The prevalence of coital incontinence can vary from 10 to 27% (Serati et al. 2009). Decreased frequency of sexual activity can also be the consequence of fear of leakage, wearing pads during the night or feeling unattractive. Incontinence was shown to have a negative effect on sexual function in 0.6–64% (Hendrix et al. 2002; Shaw 2002) of women.

5.11 Confounding Factors

5.11.1 Menopause

Several menopause-related changes in sexual function occur that have been described in the literature: diminished sexual responsiveness, dyspareunia, decreased sexual activity and decrease in sexual desire. The postmenopausal ovary has been shown to be responsible for up to 50% of the testosterone believed to be associated with libido. Androgen production by the ovary may not cease until 5 years after menopause. Many clinicians believe that a combination of both oestrogen and testosterone is required to improve female sexual function.

5.11.2 Advancing Age

Older women may not be sexually active for a variety of reasons other than urogenital prolapse. Although 60% of 60- to 69-year olds with a partner have regular coitus, many older women are widows without the possibility of having a sex life with a partner (Tannenbaum et al. 2006).

With increasing age, women often develop medical diseases and take medications that affect their sex life. These may be neurological, psychiatric or other chronic diseases with impaired mobility, which affects their social and sexual life medications such as antidepressants, antipsychotics and some diuretics affect the serotonin and dopamine actions in the brain and seem to have a negative influence on libido and arousal (Rosen et al. 1999).

5.11.3 Dysfunctional Male Partner or Lack of a Partner

Erectile dysfunction is quite common amongst older men, experienced by up to 40% amongst 70-year olds (Ellerkmann et al. 2001). Memories of past negative sexual experiences, including coercive or abusive relationships and expectations of negative outcome from dyspareunia or partner sexual dysfunction all adversely impact on sexual function (Graham et al. 2004). This will be discussed in more detail in Chap. 15.

5.11.4 Pre-prolapse Sexual Dysfunction

Sexual problems have to be considered in the context of how the patient's sex life was functioning prior to becoming incontinent or having a prolapse. Person-related resources, body image, age, physical and mental well-being and partner relationship are important factors (Ellerkmann et al. 2001).

5.11.5 Post-Partum Dyspareunia

Post-partum dyspareunia is a common and under-reported disorder. After vaginal deliveries, 41% and 22% of women at 3 and 6 months, respectively, experience dyspareunia (Salonia et al. 2004). Perineal stretching, lacerations, operative vaginal delivery and episiotomy can result in sclerotic healing and resultant entry or deep dyspareunia. The post-partum period, especially in breastfeeding women, is marked by a decrease in circulating oestrogen, which can lead to vaginal dryness and dyspareunia. The psychosexual issues of the post-partum period can lead to decreased arousal and lubrication, further contributing to dyspareunia (Handa et al. 2004). Lubricants are the typical first-line treatment. Treatment of dyspareunia specifically associated with perineal trauma during childbirth is lacking robust evidence. Post-partum pelvic organ prolapse is usually managed by physiotherapy and pessaries.

Anecdotally a change in sexual positions to minimize deeper penetration may also reduce collisional dyspareunia. Women who have persistent post-partum dyspareunia associated with identifiable perineal defects or scarring may benefit from revision perineoplasty, although this is usually reserved for significant anatomic distortions (Lukacz et al. 2007).

5.12 Assessment of POP

The aim of POP assessment is to accurately diagnose the compartment as well as extent of POP and to rule out any complications such as erosions or ulcerations. Examination should be ideally done in supine and standing position, with an empty bladder and rectum. There are several methods used to quantify POP, one of the most popular method is the Prolapse Quantification System (POP-Q) of the

International Continence Society (Bump et al. 1996). There are six defined points for measurement in the POPQ system—Aa, Ba, C, D, Ap, Bp and three others landmarks: GH, TVL and PB. Each is measured in centimetres above or proximal to the hymen (negative number) or centimetres below or distal to the hymen (positive number) with the plane of the hymen being defined as zero (0). Three other measurements are taken: the vaginal length at rest, the genital hiatus (gh) from the middle of the urethral meatus to the posterior hymenal ring and the perineal body (pb) from the posterior aspect of the genital hiatus to the mid-anal opening.

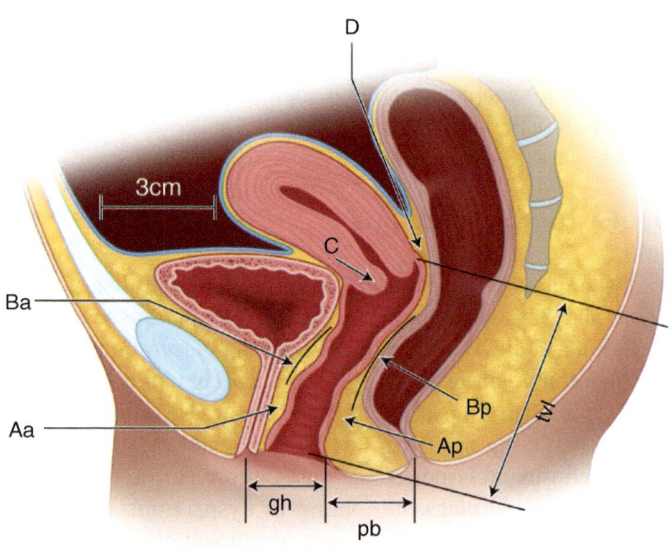

anterior wall	anterior wall	cervix or cuff
Aa	Ba	C
genital hiatus	perineal body	total vaginal length
gh	pb	tvl
posterior wall	posterior wall	posterior fornix
Ap	Bp	D

Prolapse assessment using the continence society POP-Q-Q

5.13   Investigations in POP

The diagnosis of POP is by clinical assessment; however, it is useful to perform some baseline tests to rule out bladder dysfunction, such as:

- MSU
- Urodynamics is highly recommended for women who desire interventional treatment (Abrams et al. 2005)
- Ultrasound post void residual
- CT Urogram and renal USS where upper tract involvement suspected

If bowel dysfunction is suspected, other tests such as endo anal ultrasound scan, anorectal manometry, defecating proctogram or transit studies may be required, although these are not routinely performed.

5.14   Effect of Therapeutic Interventions

Urogenital prolapse may be managed conservatively using either pelvic floor muscle training or the use of vaginal pessaries. It may also be managed surgically, and there are a large number of surgical procedures commonly used to treat pelvic floor prolapse. Each of these interventions has the potential to improve sexual function to varying degrees and with varying levels of evidence to support their use. Equally, some of these interventions may have deleterious effects on sexual function.

5.14.1 Coping Strategies

The presence of a POP can lead to "collisional dyspareunia" which can be alleviated to an extent by using certain sexual positions. The National Association for Continence advises women to:

- AVOID: Standing, 'cowgirl' or 'reverse cowgirl' [where the woman is sitting on top]. Gravity can increase the pressure on the pelvic floor in these positions.
- TRY: Modified missionary position, with the woman lying on her back with a pillow under the pelvic with her partner on top. From behind: woman lying flat on her stomach or in a supported kneeling position, with the partner entering the vagina from behind.

5.14.2 Pelvic Floor Muscle Training

PFMT is often considered as the first-line in management of urogenital prolapse. It may be the only intervention used, or as an adjunct to other options. Individualised PFMT for women with prolapse is offered by specialist women's health physiotherapists (Hagen et al. 2004). PFMT includes teaching pelvic floor exercises, vaginal examination and provision of advice regarding lifestyle changes. It may also include the use of biofeedback or neuromuscular electrical stimulation.

Although there is clear evidence that PFMT is effective in the treatment of urinary incontinence (Hay-Smith and Dumoulin 2006), similar evidence of the clinical and cost-effectiveness of PFMT in the management of prolapse is lacking. Although some studies have demonstrated the benefit of PFMT in urogenital prolapse, these have used anatomical objective cure, based on POP-Q as their primary outcome measure, patient QoL or a general measure of patient satisfaction. Sexual function has not been specifically assessed or reported in these trials (Hagen et al. 2009; Ghroubi et al. 2008). Few studies have looked at the relationship between PFMT and effect on urogenital prolapse in terms of sexual function, and the results have been conflicting (Borello et al. 2007; Braekken et al. 2015); however, PFMT has been shown to be an effective treatment for female sexual dysfunction (Borello et al. 2007; Lowenstein et al. 2010).

Given the plethora of evidence to support the use of PFMT in female sexual dysfunction as well in urogenital prolapse, it would seem sensible to continue with PFMT as the first-line option despite any clear evidence of benefit specifically in terms of sexual dysfunction in this group.

5.14.3 Pessaries

Currently vaginal pessaries are mainly used as a first-line treatment option for those patients who are either unfit for or unwilling to undergo surgery, those who wish to retain fertility or as interim relief prior to surgery and those who prefer to avoid surgery (Bash 2000). Recent evidence would suggest that more women with symptomatic prolapse would opt for pessaries rather than surgery as initial management, if offered the choice (Kapoor et al. 2009). At present there is a paucity of data on the effects of pessaries on sexual function and pelvic organ-specific symptoms during treatment with pessaries.

Some prospective studies suggest that vaginal pessaries do not interfere negatively with sexual activity and may even improve sexual function (Kuhn et al. 2009), sexual satisfaction as well as frequency of sexual activity (Fernando et al. 2006). In addition, a trial comparing the effectiveness of pessaries and surgery in women with symptomatic pelvic organ prolapse found similar improvement in urinary, bowel, sexual function and quality of life parameters using both interventions (Abdool et al. 2010).

Traditionally, physicians have considered sexual activity to be a relative contraindication to long-term pessary treatment (Cundiff et al. 2000). However, evidence suggests that sexually active women are more likely to continue wearing their pessary than women who were not sexually active, suggesting that long-term pessary use is acceptable to sexually active women (Brincat et al. 2004).

There are several pessaries available on the market that enable women to maintain sexual activity, and for many of these, it will not be noticeable to their partners.

Table 5.2 Guide to pessaries and suitability for sexual activity (Rantell 2019)

Functionality	Type of Pessary
Allow penetrative coitus whilst in situ	Ring, dish, Shaatz
Can be removed for penetrative coitus	Ring with/without support Dish with/without support Inflatoball, cube/tandem cube Gehrung
Do not allow penetrative coitus	Popy/shelf, donut, Gellhorn Hodge with/without support

If, however, the woman or their partner finds the pessary uncomfortable or obstructing during intercourse, women can be trained to remove and reinsert their pessary as necessary. The evidence suggests that, for those women who are sexually active with their pessaries in situ, they are happy and continue with this form of management in the long term (Rantell 2019).

Not all pessaries are suitable for women with POP who are sexually active. The following table (Table 5.2) details the different types of pessaries and if they are compatible with sexual activity:

Whilst considering the use of the cube, or inflatoball pessary, it must be kept in mind that these need to be self-managed. They require to be removed and cleaned on a daily basis, which requires level of manual dexterity. In addition, the inflatoball is not suitable in those with a latex allergy. Patient compliance is key with these types of pessaries as failure to remove the pessaries daily can lead to increased infection, discomfort and excoriation to the vagina. In those women who are sexually active without vaginal penetration, any pessary which is deemed to be ideal on an individualised basis may be used.

As pessaries and surgery would appear to have similar beneficial effects whilst pessaries avoid the risks of failure rates and associated increased morbidity and mortality, conservative treatment with vaginal pessaries should be discussed with all patients with urogenital prolapse, including those with sexual dysfunction. It is important to remember that long-term pessary use is not free from complications. Up to 56% of patients using pessaries long term are likely to report some complication, including bleeding, extrusion, severe vaginal discharge, pain and constipation (Sarma et al. 2009). Therefore all women opting for this treatment option should be fully informed about the risks and benefits and the importance of regular change of pessary.

5.14.4 Surgical Intervention

Surgery is often the definitive treatment for urogenital prolapse, and the lifetime risk of needing surgery is 11%, with 29.2% requiring repeat surgery (Olsen et al. 1997b). Data reporting sexual function following surgical repair are limited and conflicting. Some studies have shown an improvement (Weber et al. 2000; Rogers et al. 2006; Ghezzi et al. 2005; Srikrishna et al. 2010) whilst others have suggested a deterioration in sexual function (Mazouni et al. 2004; Helstrom and Nilsson 2005).

Pelvic surgery to correct prolapse may affect sexual function for a number of reasons including narrowed vaginal canal, poor lubrication and fear of urinary incontinence.

Vaginal dissection has been implicated in pelvic floor neuropathy affecting the pudendal nerve, which subsequently affects vaginal sensation and orgasm. Hysterectomy has been associated with sexual dysfunction, including dyspareunia as well as anorgasmia (Rhodes et al. 1999). It had been thought that removal of the cervix may alter the upper portion of the vaginal canal causing a neuropathy, although recent studies have shown that conservation of the cervix by performing a subtotal hysterectomy does not confer advantages over total hysterectomy as far as pelvic organ function is concerned. There is now considerable evidence that simple abdominal or vaginal hysterectomy does not adversely affect sexual function (Thakar and Sultan 2005). Another possible cause for dyspareunia is poor oestrogenisation of the vaginal epithelium in those women who undergo surgical menopause at the time of a hysterectomy. Therefore, careful counselling is essential in preoperative discussions especially for premenopausal women on the need, if any, to perform concomitant oophorectomy at the time of planned hysterectomy.

Repair of the anterior compartment, particularly in the absence of synthetic mesh augmentation, has not been specifically reported to cause impaired sexual function. Some studies cite an improvement in sexual function following anterior colporrhaphy (Weber et al. 2001).

Techniques used to repair a rectocele have been implicated in the cause of postoperative dyspareunia. This has been especially noted where rectocele repair has been performed via posterior colporrhaphy involving levator plication (Kahn and Stanton 1997; Jeffcoate 1959; Haase and Skibsted 1988). Site-specific repair of rectoceles has been reported to result in less dyspareunia (Porter et al. 1999; Kenton et al. 1999). Care needs to be taken in combining anterior and posterior repair as this can cause mid-vaginal stenosis and create dyspareunia.

Vaginal vault prolapse can be corrected either by an abdominal or by a vaginal approach. Sacrospinous fixation (SSF) is the most popular vaginal procedure. Sexual function after sacrospinous fixation can be altered because of pain, vaginal narrowing or pudendal nerve injury. Several studies have cited varying impact of SSF on sexual function, reporting it as maintained, improved or worsened (Holley et al. 1996; Goldberg et al. 2001; Paraiso et al. 1996; Nieminen et al. 2003).

With regard to abdominal sacrocolpopexy, two randomised controlled studies comparing vaginal and abdominal approaches have reported conflicting results. One study found no significant difference in post-operative dyspareunia in either group, although clinically more patients reported dyspareunia in the vaginal group (Benson et al. 1996). In contrast, a study done by Maher et al. found no difference in sexual function between the two groups post-operatively (Maher et al. 2004). Of patients not sexually active preoperatively, 28 and 21% resumed sexual activity postoperatively, and preoperative dyspareunia resolved in 56 and 43% in the abdominal and vaginal groups, respectively. Dyspareunia developed de novo in two women in the abdominal and three women in the vaginal group.

The use of synthetic mesh augmentation at the time of repair has also been a subject of debate with some studies suggesting increased levels of persistent dyspareunia in 50% of sexually active women when compared to native tissue repair (Blandon et al. 2009). However, a randomised controlled trial comparing vaginal repair augmented by mesh with traditional colporrhaphy for the treatment of pelvic organ prolapse found similar rates of de novo dyspareunia in both groups. [16.7% in the mesh group and 15.2% in the no mesh group at 12 months] (Carey et al. 2009). Similarly, another randomised study involving 97 patients randomised to colporrhaphy with no mesh and 105 with mesh found that dyspareunia was statistically significantly lower in the mesh group (Nieminen et al. 2008). More recently, a review into outcomes following surgical repair found that, although most patients experience improvements in their sexual response, surgical approaches involving abdominal or transvaginal mesh may result in a decline in sexual function and worsening dyspareunia (Shatkin-Margolis et al. 2017).

5.15 Conclusion

Sexual well-being is an important aspect of women's health, and dysfunction can lead to a decrease in quality of life and affect personal relationships. Although female sexual dysfunction is a common problem especially in patients with urogenital prolapse, it has been poorly studied in the literature. Consequently, data on the prevalence of sexual dysfunction as well as effects of different therapeutic interventions are limited.

The pathophysiology of female sexual dysfunction is complex and multifactorial. It may involve several physical, social and psychological dimensions. Women with urogenital prolapse are typically older and postmenopausal, with several associated confounding factors which may have an impact on their sexual function.

The management of pelvic floor dysfunction is varied, and the impact of different interventions on sexual function has been poorly studied. Most therapies have the potential to improve sexual function, although some are also known to cause sexual difficulties. It is therefore important for all trials on therapeutic interventions in urogenital prolapse to include functional outcome assessment, including sexual function. This will allow clinicians to counsel individual women with urogenital prolapse on the benefits and potential disadvantages of each therapy on sexual function.

References

Abdool Z, Thakar R, Sultan AH, Oliver RS (2010) Prospective evaluation of outcome of vaginal pessaries versus surgery in women with symptomatic pelvic organ prolapse. Int Urogynecol J Pelvic Floor Dysfunct 22(3):273–278

Abrams P, Andersson KE, Brubaker L (2005) Recommendations of the International Scientific Committee: evaluation and treatment of urinary incontinence, pelvic organ prolapse and faecal incontinence. Health Publications, Paris, pp 1589–1630

Barber MD, Visco AG, Wyman JF, Fantl JA, Bump RC (2002) Sexual function in women with urinary incontinence and pelvic organ prolapse. Obstet Gynecol 99:281–289

Bash KL (2000) Review of vaginal pessaries. Obstet Gynecol Surv 55:455–460

Benson JT, Lucente V, McClellan E (1996) Vaginal versus abdominal reconstructive surgery for the treatment of pelvic support defects: a prospective randomized study with long-term outcome evaluation. Am J Obstet Gynecol 175(6):1418–1421

Berman JR, Berman LA, Werbin TJ, Flaherty EE, Leahy NM, Goldstein I (1999) Clinical evaluation of female sexual function: effects of age and estrogen status on subjective and physiologic sexual responses. Int J Impot Res Suppl 1:S31–S38

Blandon RE, Gebhart JB, Trabuco EC, Klingele CJ (2009) Complications from vaginally placed mesh in pelvic reconstructive surgery. Int Urogynecol J Pelvic Floor Dysfunct 20(5):523–531. https://doi.org/10.1007/s00192-009-0818-9. Epub 2009 Feb 10. PMID: 19209374

Borello-France DF, Handa VL, Brown MB, Goode P, Kreder K, Scheufele LL, Weber AM, Pelvic Floor Disorders Network (2007) Pelvic-floor muscle function in women with pelvic organ prolapse. Phys Ther. 87(4):399–407

Braekken IH, Majida M, Ellström Engh M, Bø K (2015) Can pelvic floor muscle training improve sexual function in women with pelvic organ prolapse? A randomized controlled trial. J Sex Med 12(2):470–480. https://doi.org/10.1111/jsm.12746. Epub 2014 Nov 17

Brincat C, Kenton K, Pat Fitzgerald M, Brubaker L (2004) Sexual activity predicts continued pessary use. Am J Obstet Gynecol. 191(1):198–200

Bump RC, Mattiasson A, Bø K et al (1996) The standardization of terminology of female pelvic organ prolapse and pelvic floor dysfunction. Am J Obstet Gynecol 175:10–17

Carey M, Higgs P, Goh J, Lim J, Leong A, Krause H, Cornish A (2009) Vaginal repair with mesh versus colporrhaphy for prolapse: a randomised controlled trial. BJOG 116(10):1380–1386

Cundiff GW, Weidner AC, Visco AG, Bump RC, Addison WA (2000) A survey of pessary use by members of the American urogynecologic society. Obstet Gynecol **95**:931–935

Dennerstein L, Alexander JL, Kotz K (2003) The menopause and sexual functioning: a review of the population-based studies. Annu Rev Sex Res 14:64–82

Digesu GA, Khullar V, Cardozo L, Robinson D, Salvatore S (2005) P-QoL: a validated questionnaire to assess the symptoms and quality of life of women with urogenital prolapse. Int Urogynecol J 16:176–181

Ellerkmann RM, Cundiff GW, Melick CF et al (2001) Correlation of symptoms with location and severity of pelvic organ prolapse. Am J Obstet Gynecol 185:1332–1337

Fernando RJ, Thakar R, Sultan AH, Shah SM, Jones PW (2006) Effect of vaginal pessaries on symptoms associated with pelvic organ prolapse. Obstet Gynecol. 108(1):93–99

Ghezzi F, Serati M, Cromi A, Uccella S, Triacca P, Bolis P (2005) Impact of tension-free vaginal tape on sexual function: results of a prospective study. Int Urogynecol J Pelvic Floor Dysfunct 17:54–59

Ghroubi S, Kharrat O, Chaari M, Ben Ayed B, Guermazi M, Elleuch MH (2008) Effect of conservative treatment in the management of low-degree urogenital prolapse. Ann Readapt Med Phys 51:96–102

Giarenis I, Robinson D (2014) Prevention and management of pelvic organ prolapse. F1000Prime Rep 6:77. https://doi.org/10.12703/P6-77. PMID: 25343034; PMCID: PMC4166938

Goldberg RP, Tomezsko JE, Winkler HA et al (2001) Anterior or posterior sacrospinous vaginal vault suspension: long-term anatomic and functional evaluation. Obstet Gynecol 98(2):199–204

Graham CA, Sanders SA, Milhausen RR, McBride KR (2004) Turning on and turning off: a focus group study of the factors that affect women's sexual arousal. Arch Sex Behav 33(6):527–538

Gyhagen M, Bullarbo M, Nielsen TF, Milsom I (2013) Prevalence and risk factors for pelvic organ prolapse 20 years after childbirth: a national cohort study in singleton primiparae after vaginal or caesarean delivery. BJOG 120(2):152–160

Haase P, Skibsted L (1988) Influence of operations for stress incontinence and/or genital descensus on sexual life. Acta Obstet Gynecol Scand 67(7):659–661

Hagen S, Stark D, Cattermole D (2004) A United Kingdom-wide survey of physiotherapy practice in the treatment of pelvic organ prolapse. Physiotherapy 90(1):19–26

Hagen S, Stark D, Glazener C, Sinclair L, Ramsay I (2009) A randomized controlled trial of pelvic floor muscle training for stages I and II pelvic organ prolapse. Int Urogynecol J Pelvic Floor Dysfunct 20(1):45–51

Handa VL, Harvey L, Cundiff GW, Siddique SA, Kjerulff KH (2004) Sexual function among women with urinary incontinence and pelvic organ prolapse. Am J Obstet Gynecol. 191(3):751–756

Handa VL, Cundiff G, Chang HH, Helzlsouer KJ (2008) Female sexual function and pelvic floor disorders. Obstet Gynecol 111(5):1037–1038

Hartmann U, Philippsohn S, Heiser K, Ruffer-Hesse C (2004) Low sexual desire in midlife and older women: personality factors, psychosocial development, present sexuality. Menopause 11:726–740

Haylen et al (2016) An International Urogynecological Association (IUGA)/International Continence Society (ICS) Joint Report on the Terminology for Female Pelvic Organ Prolapse (POP). Neurourol Urodyn 35:137–168

Hay-Smith EJC, Dumoulin C (2006) Pelvic floor muscle training versus no treatment, or inactive control treatments, for urinary incontinence in women. Cochrane Database Syst Rev (1):CD005654. https://doi.org/10.1002/14651858

Helström L, Nilsson B (2005) Impact of vaginal surgery on sexuality and quality of life in women with urinary incontinence or genital descensus. Acta Obstet Gynecol Scand. 84(1): 79–84

Helstrom L, Nilsson B (2005) Impact of vaginal surgery on sexuality and quality of life in women with urinary incontinence or genital descensus. Acta Obstet Gynecol Scand 84:79–84

Hendrix SL, Clark A, Nygaard I, Aragaki A, Barnabei V, McTiernan A (2002) Pelvic organ prolapse in the Women's Health Initiative: gravity and gravidity. Am J Obstet Gynecol 186:1160–1166

Holley RL, Varner RE, Gleason BP et al (1996) Sexual function after sacrospinous ligament fixation for vaginal vault prolapse. J Reprod Med 41(5):355–358

Hunskaar S, Burgio K, Clark A et al (2005) Epidemiology of urinary and fecal incontinence and pelvic organ prolapse. In: Abrams P, Cordozo L, Koury S, Wein A (eds) Third international consultation on incontinence, 1st edn. Health Publication, Paris

Jeffcoate TN (1959) Posterior colpoperineorrhaphy. Am J Obstet Gynecol 77(3):490–502

Jelovsek JE, Barber MD (2006) Women seeking treatment for advanced pelvic organ prolapse have decreased body image and quality of life. Am J Obstet Gynecol. 194(5):1455–1461

Kahn MA, Stanton SL (1997) Posterior colporrhaphy: its effects on bowel and sexual function. Br J Obstet Gynaecol 104:82–86

Kapoor DS, Thakar R, Sultan AH, Oliver R (2009) Conservative versus surgical managment of prolapse: what dictates patient choice? Int Urogynecol J Pelvic Floor Dycfunct 20:1157–1161

Kelleher CJ, Cardozo LD, Khullar V, Salvatore S (1997) A new questionnaire to assess the quality of life of urinary incontinent women. Br J Obstet Gynaecol 104:1374–1379

Kenton K, Shott S, Brubaker L (1999) Outcome after rectovaginal fascia reattachment for rectocele repair. Am J Obstet Gynecol 181:1360–1364

Kuhn A, Bapst D, Stadlmayr W, Vits K, Mueller MD (2009) Sexual and organ function in patients with symptomatic prolapse: are pessaries helpful? Fertil Steril. 91(5):1914–1918

Laan E, van Driel E, van Lunsen RHW (2003) Sexual responses of women with sexual arousal disorder to visual sexual stimuli. Tijdschr Seksual 27:1–13

Lowenstein L, Gruenwald I, Gartman I, Vardi Y (2010) Can stronger pelvic muscle floor improve sexual function? Int Urogynecol J Pelvic Floor Dysfunct. 21(5):553–556

Lukacz ES, Whitcomb EL, Lawrence JM, Nager CW, Contreras R, Luber KM (2007) Are sexual activity and satisfaction affected by pelvic floor disorders? Analysis of a community-based survey. Am J Obstet Gynecol. 197(1):88–86

Maher CF, Qatawneh AM, Dwyer PL et al (2004) Abdominal sacral colpopexy or vaginal sacrospinous colpopexy for vaginal vault prolapse: a prospective randomized study. Am J Obstet Gynecol 190(1):20–26

Mant J, Painter R, Vessey M (1997) Epidemiology of genital prolapse: observations from the Oxford family planning association study. BJOG 104:579–585

Mazouni C, Karsenty G, Bretelle F, Bladou F, Gamerre M, Serment G (2004) Urinary complications and sexual function after the tension-free vaginal tape procedure. Acta Obstet Gynecol Scand 83:955–961

Moalli PA, Ivy SJ, Meyn LA, Zyczynski HM (2003) Risk factors associated with pelvic floor disorders in women undergoing surgical repair. Obstet Gynecol 101:869–874

Moroni RM, Alves da Silva Lara L, CHJ F, de Mello Constantino M, Oliveira Brito LG (2019) Assessment of body image, sexual function, and attractiveness in women with genital prolapse: a cross-sectional study with validation of the Body Image in the Pelvic Organ Prolapse (BIPOP) Questionnaire. J Sex Med 16(1):126–136. https://doi.org/10.1016/j.jsxm.2018.11.005

Nieminen K, Huhtala H, Heinonen PK (2003) Anatomic and functional assessment and risk factors of recurrent prolapse after vaginal sacrospinous fixation. Acta Obstet Gynecol Scand 82(5):471–478

Nieminen K, Hiltunen R, Heiskanen E, Takala T, Niemi K, Merikari M, Heinonen PK (2008) Symptom resolution and sexual function after anterior vaginal wall repair with or without polypropylene mesh. Int Urogynecol J Pelvic Floor Dysfunct 19(12):1611–1616

Olsen AL, Smith VJ, Bergstrom JO, Colling JC, Clark AL (1997a) Epidemiology of surgically managed pelvic organ prolapse and urinary incontinence. Obstet Gynecol 89:501–506

Olsen AL, Smith VJ, Bergstrom JO, Colling JC, Clark AL (1997b) Epidemiology of surgically managed pelvic organ prolapse and urinary incontinence. Obstet Gynaecol 89(4):501–506

Paraiso MFR, Ballard LA, Walters M et al (1996) Pelvic support defects and visceral and sexual function in women treated with sacrospinous ligament suspension and pelvic reconstruction. Am J Obstet Gynecol 175:1423–1431

Pauls RN, Segal JL, Andre Silva W, Kleeman SD, Karram MM (2006) Sexual function in patients presenting to a urogynecology practice. Int Urogynecol J Pelvic Floor Dysfunct 17:576–580

Porter WE, Steele A, Walsh P et al (1999) The anatomic and functional outcomes of defect specific rectocele repairs. Am J Obstet Gynecol 181:1353–1359

Rantell A (2019) Vaginal pessaries for pelvic organ prolapse and their impact on sexual function. Sex Med Rev. 7(4):597–603. https://doi.org/10.1016/j.sxmr.2019.06.002. Epub 2019 Aug 2. Review

Rhodes JC, Kjerulff KH, Langenberg PW et al (1999) Hysterectomy and sexual functioning. JAMA 282:1934–1947

Rogers RG, Kammerer-Doak D, Darrow A et al (2006) Does sexual function change after surgery for stress urinary incontinence and/or pelvic organ prolapse? A multicenter prospective study. Am J Obstet Gynecol 195:e1–e4

Rogers RG, Pauls RN, Thakar R, Morin M, Kuhn A, Petri E, Fatton B, Whitmore K, Kinsberg S, Lee J (2018) An International Urogynecological Association (IUGA)/International Continence Society (ICS) joint report on the terminology for the assessment of sexual health of women with pelvic floor dysfunction. Neurourol Urodyn 37(4):1220–1240

Rosen R, Lane R, Menza M (1999) Effects of SSRIs on sexual function: a critical review. J Clin Psychopharmacol 19:67–85

Salonia A, Zanni G, Nappi RE et al (2004) Sexual dysfunction is common in women with lower urinary tract symptoms and urinary incontinence: results of a cross-sectional study. Eur Urol 45:642–648

Sarma S, Ying T, Moore KH (2009) Long-term vaginal ring pessary use: discontinuation rates and adverse events. BJOG. 116(13):1715–1721

Sarrel P, Dobay B, Wiita B (1998) Estrogen and estrogen– androgen replacement in postmenopausal women dissatisfied with estrogen only therapy: sexual behaviour and neuroendocrine responses. J Reprod Med 43:847–855

Serati M, Salvatore S, Uccella S, Nappi RE, Bolis P (2009) Female urinary incontinence during intercourse: a review on an understudied problem for women's sexuality. J Sex Med. 6(1):40–48

Shatkin-Margolis A, Pauls R (2017) "Sexual function after prolapse repair." Curr Opin Obstet Gynecol 29:343–348

Shaw C (2002) A systematic review of the literature on the prevalence of sexual impaiment in women with urinary incontinence and the prevalence of urinary leakage during sexual activity. Eur Urol 42:432–440

Slieker-ten HMCP, Vierhout M, Bloembergen H, Schoenmaker G (2004) Distribution of pelvic organ prolapse in a general population: prevalence, severity, aetiology and relation with function of pelvic floor muscles. In: Abstract presented at the joint meeting of ICS and IUGA, Paris, 25–27 Aug 2004

Srikrishna S, Robinson D, Cardozo L, Gonzalez J (2010) Can sex survive pelvic floor surgery? Int Urogynecol J 21(11):1313–1319. https://doi.org/10.1007/s00192-010-1198-x. Epub 2010 Jun 25

Suckling J, Lethaby A, Kennedy R (2003) Local oestrogen for vaginal atrophy in postmenopausal women. Cochrane Database Syst Rev (4):CD001500

Swift SE (2000) The distribution of pelvic organ support in a population of female subjects seen for routine gynaecological health care. Am J Obstet Gynecol 183:277–285

Swift SE, Woodman P, O'Boyle A et al (2005a) Pelvic Organ Support Study (POSST): the distribution, clinical definition and epidemiology of pelvic organ support defects. Am J Obstet Gynecol 192:795–806

Swift S, Woodman P, O'Boyle A et al (2005b) Pelvic Organ Support Study (POSST): the distribution, clinical definition, and epidemiologic condition of pelvic organ support defects. Am J Obstet Gynecol 192:795–806

Tannenbaum C, Corcos J, Assalian P (2006) The relationship between sexual activity and urinary incontinence in older women. J Am Geriatr Soc 54:1220–1224

Teunissen D, Bosch WVD, Weel CV, Largo-Janssen T (2006) "It can always happen": the impact of urinary incontinence on elderly men and women. Scand J Prim Health Care 24:166–173

Thakar R, Sultan AH (2005) Hysterectomy and pelvic organ dysfunction. Best Pract Res Clin Obstet Gynaecol. 19(3):403–418. Epub 2005 Feb 12

Verbeek M, Hayward L (2019) Pelvic floor dysfunction and its effect on quality of sexual life. Sex Med Rev. 7(4):559–564. https://doi.org/10.1016/j.sxmr.2019.05.007. Epub 2019 Jul 24. Review

Weber AM, Walters MD, Schover LR, Mitchinson A (1995) Sexual function in women with uterovaginal prolapse and urinary incontinence. Obstet Gynecol. 85(4):483–487

Weber AM, Walters MD, Piedmonte MR (2000) Sexual function and vaginal anatomy in women before and after surgery for pelvic organ prolapse and urinary incontinence. Am J Obstet Gynecol 182:1610–1615

Weber AM, Walters MD, Piedmonte MR, Ballard LA (2001) Anterior colporrhaphy: a randomized trial of three surgical techniques. Am J Obstet Gynecol 185(6):1299–1304

The Impact of Recurrent Urinary Tract Infections on Sexual Function

6

Georgina Baines and Cathy Davis

6.1 Definition of Urinary Tract Infection

A urinary tract infection (UTI) is the presence of significant bacteria and pus in the urine, along with increased bladder sensation, urgency, frequency, dysuria, urgency urinary incontinence and/or pain (Naber et al. 2001). In hospital medicine, UTI is significant, as it can be a precursor to infection of the upper urinary tracts (pyelonephritis). With an anatomically normal urinary tract, the progression from UTI to pyelonephritis is 2% (Christiaens et al. 2002).

6.2 Symptoms

For most women, it is not the risk of ascending infection that is troublesome, but the symptoms of the UTI. Many women will describe the symptoms experienced as 'cystitis'. The most common symptoms are frequency of urine and dysuria, but others encountered are suprapubic pain, haematuria, urethritis or vaginitis and feeling generally unwell (Bent et al. 2002; Stamm et al. 1982). As the risk of ascending infection is low, the main aim of diagnosis and treatment is amelioration of these symptoms.

Symptoms of UTI
Passing urine frequently
Pain on passing urine

G. Baines (✉)
King's College Hospital, London, UK
e-mail: g.baines1@nhs.net

C. Davis
Urogynaecology Department, King's College Hospital, London, UK
e-mail: cathydavis@nhs.net

© Springer Nature Switzerland AG 2021
A. Rantell (ed.), *Sexual Function and Pelvic Floor Dysfunction*,
https://doi.org/10.1007/978-3-030-63843-6_6

Symptoms of UTI
Pain in the lower abdomen
Irritation of the urethra or vagina
Feeling unwell
Smelly urine

6.3   Diagnosis

UTI can be difficult to diagnose but it is generally accepted that a positive urine culture is indicative of UTI. Urine is cultured in a laboratory and the predominant organisms identified. Significant growth is defined as identification of a single organism $\geq 10^5$ colony forming units (CFU) in a specimen of urine obtained from the middle of the stream of urine (Naber et al. 2001). Bacteria grown at culture usually originate from the gut or vagina (Foxman 2010).

These diagnostic criteria are historical and are based on increasing risk of ascending infection rather than impact of symptoms on the patient. Because of this, some clinicians feel that these criteria may not be a sensitive enough tool for diagnosing troublesome UTI. It has been shown that if a more sensitive test to look for bacterial DNA in the urine (polymerase chain reaction; PCR), 80% of women with symptoms of UTI and a negative culture will be positive for a uropathogen (Heytens et al. 2017). We may need to rethink how UTI is diagnosed in women.

Culturing urine can take a number of days, so in order to guide rapid treatment a bedside test widely utilised is the urine dipstick. The presence of nitrites in the urine (produced by bacteria) has a positive predictive value of 96% but a sensitivity of 35–57% (Masajtis-Zagajewska and Nowicki 2017). When the presence of white blood cells (leukocytes) and nitrites are used, the positive predictive value is 66.7% and the negative predictive value is 77.4% (Najeeb et al. 2015). These figures demonstrate the imperfect nature of urine dipstick in diagnosing UTI in women. The dipstick is also not reliable in women over the age of 65 and those with catheters in situ. In these cases, a urine culture should be sent.

Symptoms correlate well with diagnosis and it has been shown that when frequency and dysuria are reported, there is a 90% risk of there being a UTI diagnosed (Bent et al. 2002). Therefore the National Institute for Clinical Excellence (NICE) advises treatment for presumed UTI when the patient reports symptoms along with a urine dipstick positive for nitrites (the result of reduction of nitrates by bacteria) (Excellence NIfHaC 2018). Pyuria on microscopy or dipstick is widely used as a surrogate marker for UTI, but its presence or absence may not correlate with infection (Kupelian et al. 2013). NICE recommends that if the dipstick is positive for leukocytes and blood then UTI is likely, but if only leukocytes then other diagnoses are equally as likely (Excellence NIfHaC 2018). They advised that urine dipstick should not be used to diagnose UTI in patients who have a catheter in situ. The presence of a catheter can cause an increase in leukocytes in the urine in the absence of infection, so increasing false-positive diagnoses.

The finding of blood on urine dipstick or microscopic haematuria can be indicative of serious underlying pathology such as urolithiasis (stone formation), malignancy or renal disease and appropriate investigations should be undertaken (Linder et al. 2018).

Once UTI is diagnosed, we must consider further investigations. If anatomical abnormality of the urinary tract is suspected, imaging in the form of ultrasound or enhanced CT can be useful. Cystoscopy with or without biopsy can be used to identify inter-vesical lesions and inflammation.

When to send a urine culture?
Women over 65 years
Pregnant women
Persistent symptoms not improving with antibiotics
Recurrent UTI
Catheterised women
If there are risk factors for complicated UTI (e.g. renal failure, abnormal anatomy)
Visible or non-visible haematuria

6.4 Definition of Recurrent Urinary Tract Infection (rUTI)

Recurrent UTIs (rUTI)s are symptomatic infections following the complete resolution of a previous infection (Hooton 2001). Once a woman has had a UTI, she has a 25% chance of suffering a recurrence of infection in the next 3–6 months (Foxman 1990). This is more common in women over the age of 55 years, with 53% of these women reporting a recurrence in the following 12 months (compared to 36% in those aged 18–55) (Ikäheimo et al. 1996). RUTI are defined as >2 infections over a 6-month period or 3 infections over 12 months with complete resolution for at least 2 weeks (Foxman 1990).

Some women may suffer from symptoms more suggestive of one persistent infection rather than multiple recurrent UTIs, which may benefit from similar management strategies to rUTI.

6.5 Uropathogens

UTIs are caused by a wide range of organisms which are termed 'uropathogens' when causing infection in the urinary tract. They can be gram-negative or gram-positive bacteria or even fungi.

Escherichia Coli is the most commonly identified uropathogen in complicated (65%) and uncomplicated (75%) UTIs. The other uropathogens implicated are *Klebsiella pneumoniae*, *Staphylococcus saprophyticus* and *Enterococcus faecalis. Of interest, candida is the causative organism in 7% of complicated UTIs but only 1% of uncomplicated infections (*Flores-Mireles et al. 2015*).*

E. coli is demonstrated in up to 80% of cases in Europe (Carlsen et al. 2019; Kornfält Isberg et al. 2019; Alós 2005). *E. coli* is the most prevalent bacteria in the human gastrointestinal tract (Sahoo et al. 2012) and when this is transferred to the urinary tract, the bacteria can become pathological causing the symptoms of UTI. Women have a much shorter urethra compared to men, thus allowing the retrograde passage of uropathogens more easily which explains why men do not tend to suffer from UTIs as much. Women who suffer from rUTI are more likely to have rectal *E. coli* diagnosed than those without (Stamey and Sexton 1975). It is felt that any activity, which facilitates the passage of bacteria between the anus and the urinary tract, may cause or exacerbate UTIs. Sexual intercourse is an obvious factor to cause this, and it has been shown that it is a risk factor for rUTI (Scholes et al. 2000). Whilst *E. coli* is the most commonly implicated bacteria, there are many others that can cause problematic infection of the urinary tract, many of these also from the gram-negative *Enterobacteriaceae* family (Kodner and Thomas Gupton 2010).

When thinking about UTI in the context of sex, an important organism to mention is *Ureaplasma urealyticum*. It belongs to the *Mycoplasmataceae* family of bacteria, which lack a cell wall and live inside the host cells. *Ureaplasma* has been shown to be present in 33% of women attending with lower urinary tract symptoms (Latthe et al. 2008). It is a sexually transmitted infection and can also cause pelvic inflammatory disease and subsequent infertility.

6.6   Pathogenesis of rUTI

UTIs can be classified as uncomplicated or complicated. Complicated UTIs are those associated with factors that compromise the urinary tract or immune system. These can include abnormal anatomy of the urinary tract (including calculi), immunosuppression, renal failure or indwelling catheters (Flores-Mireles et al. 2015).

Uncomplicated UTIs are those occurring in women without these risk factors who are otherwise healthy. In this group of women, the transfer of uropathogens from the rectum to the urethra is a key action in the causation of repeated infections. However, it has been shown that following an initial UTI and antibiotic treatment, 77% of subsequent infections are with the identical strain of *E. coli* (Ejrnæs 2011). This implies an alternative mechanism where the primary infection is not completely cleared. This is supported by data showing that antibacterial perineal washing does not reduce the risk of rUTI (Cass and Ireland 1985). There is most likely two mechanisms by which women suffer rUTI; repeat infection from gut commensals and chronic cystitis flares.

6.7   Prevalence

UTI is a common condition that one in three women will experience by the age of 24 and half of all women will suffer at least one UTI during their lifetime (Foxman 2003). UTI is generally managed in primary care and is the most commonly diagnosed infection in this setting (Car 2006). UTI therefore accounts for a significant proportion of antibiotics prescribed by general practitioners (Foxman 2003).

The incidence of UTI in women increases with age, with the exception of a spike in younger women aged 14–24 years (Schmiemann et al. 2010). This coincides with a peak in sexual activity, particularly between the ages of 18 and 39 (Medina and Castillo-Pino 2019).

6.8   Risk Factors for UTI

Looking at all causes of UTIs, it is clear that iatrogenic causes are common. Hospital-acquired urinary tract infections are a leading cause of health-care infections in geriatrics, psychiatry and obstetrics and gynaecology. These are primarily caused by the use of indwelling urinary catheters (Gardner et al. 2014) and are therefore classified as complicated UTIs.

Obstruction or abnormal anatomy of the urinary tract can cause urinary stasis or ureteric reflux, allowing establishment of UTI and suboptimal clearance of infection. Likewise, voiding dysfunction with a significant residual volume (>100 ml) is associated with UTI. Urinary tract stones may serve as a focus for the formation of infection (Tandogdu and Wagenlehner 2016).

Women with diabetes demonstrate an impairment in innate and acquired immune function which can make them more susceptible to any infection including UTIs (Tanaka 2008). Equally, women with renal failure and those on immunosuppressive medication are less able to mount a defence to bacteria in the urinary tract.

It is thought that some behavioural or hygiene practices may be associated with an increased risk of rUTI, some of which may be supported by evidence and/or anecdote. It is clear that increasing water intake can reduce UTI (Popkin et al. 2010); however, there is no evidence to suggest that this can help rUTI (Scholes et al. 2000). Women who regularly use spermicidal agents or those on the combined oral contraceptive pill are at an increased risk of rUTI (Scholes et al. 2000). It is known that voiding less than three times a day is associated with higher risk of UTI (Nielsen and Walter 1994) and frequent voiding can be protective (Su et al. 2009). Toileting habits such as the use of feminine/baby wipes can be associated with UTI (Crann et al. 2018).

A recent study showed some evidence for several modifiable behavioural patterns which influence frequency of rUTI. They reported that wiping back to front, not voiding within 15 min of intercourse, not drinking water after intercourse and using soap to wash genitals were all associated with an increased risk of UTI (Al Demour and Ababneh 2018).

Recurrent UTI can be triggered by intercourse and increased frequency of intercourse increases risk of UTI, as does having a new sexual partner in the preceding 12 months (Scholes et al. 2000). We know that a majority of uropathogens originate in the gastrointestinal tract. Vaginal penetrative intercourse can exacerbate transfer of these bacteria from the gastrointestinal tract to the urethra.

Over recent years, trends in sexual behaviour have been changing. Although the number of occasions of sexual activity in the last month has decreased between 1990 and 2010 (6.1 to 4.8), the number of women who had anal intercourse in the preceding year had more than doubled, from 6.5 to 15% in the same time period (Mercer et al. 2013). It is likely that anal intercourse increases the risk of bacterial transfer, particularly if vaginal penetration occurs subsequently.

6.9   Impact on Quality of Life

There are a paucity of data on the impact of rUTI on quality of life, but that available would suggest it is associated with mental stress (Wagenlehner et al. 2018; Ennis et al. 2018; Ellis and Verma 2000), and that patients would like their physicians to have a better understanding of their symptoms and the impact they have on their lives (Moskowitz and Lee 2018).

The GESPRIT study aimed to assess the personal and economic burden of rUTI in Europe. An online questionnaire was sent to women complaining of rUTI and completed by 1275 women who currently had an acute infection and 666 women who had suffered one in the previous 4 weeks. Eighty percent of women reported having received antibiotics to treat their infection and the majority found behavioural changes ineffective. On average, there were 3 days of sick leave taken for UTI symptoms with 3.74 days of limited activity reported in each year (Wagenlehner et al. 2018).

The unpredictable, acute presentation of UTI can cause distress and anxiety in the patient, and treating the acute infection with antibiotics is often not sufficient to prevent this (Schmiemann et al. 2010). Reducing the occurrence of UTI may help reduce the emotional burden.

In an observational study of 575 patients affected by rUTI, 61% exhibited some degree of depression at baseline as assessed by the *Hospital Anxiety and Depression Scale* (HADS). Following treatment with lyophilized bacterial lysate, the number of UTIs decreased by 59% with a corresponding decrease in the HADS by 32.1% (Renard et al. 2014). This shows an association between a decreasing frequency of UTI and improvements in anxiety and depression.

6.10   Treatment of UTI

The first-line of treatment for uncomplicated UTI is antibiotics. A 3-day course is usually recommended as there is better compliance, lower cost and fewer adverse reactions compared to longer courses (Warren et al. 1999). As UTI is the most prevalent infection encountered in primary care (Car 2006), it results in a high number of antibiotic prescriptions which drives resistance (Malcolm et al. 2018). In women with rUTI, urine culture results should guide antimicrobial therapy.

Ureaplasma will not be grown on typical culture so therefore PCR should be undertaken to identify the bacteria's genetic code. If this is found to be positive, a

14-day course of doxycycline is advised along with sexual contact tracing and testing.

When a woman is suffering from rUTI, behavioural modifications should be the first-line once an acute infection has been treated appropriately (Excellence NIfHaC 2018). These involve modifications to sexual activity and contraceptive use. If a woman is using diaphragms or spermicides, alternatives should be offered. As there is a lack of robust evidence on other behavioural practices (e.g. direction of wiping, pre or post-coital voiding), there is disagreement over what advice should be given to patients (Aydin et al. 2015).

Continuous prophylaxis with nightly antibiotic can reduce the frequency of UTI by 95% when compared to placebo (Nicolle and Ronald 1987). However, constant antibiotic use may drive resistance rates and be less acceptable to patients.

Post-coital prophylaxis is when the patient takes a single dose of antibiotics following sexual intercourse. This has been shown to be as effective as continuous prophylaxis and is more acceptable to patients (Hooton 2001).

Other non-antibiotic treatments include cranberry juice or tablets and D-mannose supplements. The evidence for these therapies is mixed but as they have minimal side effects, may be trialled in motivated patients.

Methenamine salts dissolve in urine to form ammonia and formaldehyde, which acts as a bactericide, sterilising the urine. A Cochrane review has shown that methenamine hippurate is effective in preventing UTI in the short term (Lee et al. 2012).

Exogenous oestrogen may be a useful treatment in postmenopausal women suffering from rUTIs. Oestrogen plays an important role in maintaining the health of the vagina and lower urinary tract. Data from a limited number of studies show that vaginal oestrogens can decrease the number of UTIs in postmenopausal women (Perrotta et al. 2008).

A promising new treatment has recently become available in Europe with the aim of modulating the immune system in women with rUTI. Uromune is a sublingual vaccine, which works by stimulating a host response against *E. coli*, *Klebsiella*, *Proteus* and *Enterococcus faecalis*. Data are lacking but a UK study showed a 78% reduction in UTIs when women are treated with the vaccine (Yang and Foley 2018).

Probiotics (e.g. *Lactobacilli*) have been used to help prevent rUTIs. The rationale for their use is that they help maintain a barrier in the lower urinary tract to prevent ascending infection from the vagina and urethra by reducing adherence of the pathogens, growth and colonisation and modulating the host defences. A Cochrane review found that there was no evidence to suggest that their use clinically decreases rate of UTI; however, they did acknowledge that the evidence available was poor (Schwenger et al. 2015).

A more invasive treatment that has been used since the 1960s involves instillation of agents into the bladder. This can be hyaluronic acid compounds, which aim to replenish the layer protecting the inside of the bladder, or more recently antibiotics. These treatments often involve prolonged courses and a requirement for the patient to be able to self-catheterise to administer the instillation or attend a clinic regularly for treatment. There are mixed results reported but generally it is accepted as an end-stage treatment.

6.11   Sexual Function

It is clear that there is a close relationship between sexual intercourse and recurrent urinary tract infections with increasing frequency of intercourse, worsening rUTI. There is little evidence to explore the effect that suffering from rUTI will have on sexual function although it is known that other lower urinary tract symptoms can have a negative effect on this (Constantine et al. 2017).

As sexual relationships and behaviour are a key-component of maintaining a good quality of life (Mercer et al. 2013), any factors that influence this may not only have an adverse effect on sexual function but on quality of life.

As sexual intercourse is a major factor in triggering UTI, especially in younger women, avoidance strategies may be taken. These can develop into fear of intercourse and subsequently vaginismus. Patients may find these problems difficult to discuss with their partner, causing emotional stress on both the patient and her partner and have a negative impact on the relationship.

Advice on sexual hygiene may help reduce the incidence of UTI by minimising transfer of bacteria. This can include washing genitals prior to intercourse, avoiding anal intercourse particularly with subsequent vaginal penetration. Voiding following sex will empty the bladder and urethra of urine and potential uropathogens (although not supported by evidence, this advice is widely given). However, although potentially helpful, these behavioural and hygiene factors may generate anxiety around sexual intercourse. Partners may not be understanding of the measures required which can cause tension in a relationship. This could also result in the patient holding the partners' hygiene habits responsible for their UTI, which will have a significant impact on the relationship.

The effects of treatment on sexual function are an important factor to consider. Prolonged courses of antibiotics may cause changes in the vaginal flora leading to candida infections. This can make intercourse uncomfortable and again avoidance strategies employed.

If more invasive treatments such as instillations are utilised, there may be stigma surrounding self-catheterisation, which could go on to, affect the woman's feelings towards sexual intercourse.

In general, there is a lack of evidence regarding the effect of rUTI on sexual function in women. It seems evident however that there is a considerable link between not only the cause of UTIs but also the treatments and sex.

When caring for these women in primary and secondary care, we should be mindful of the fact that sexual function may be a sensitive topic for the patient and may even be her reason for seeking help. In routine practice, we advise the behavioural and sexual changes listed below, but we must remember that very few of these are supported by high quality evidence and that we may be having a detrimental impact on the patient's quality of life.

Behavioural changes advised
Wipe perineum front to back
Do not use perfumed wipes or soaps/"feminine hygiene" products
Take showers not baths if possible
Avoid tights/tight trousers
Avoid bladder irritants, e.g. caffeine
Avoid constipation
Void regularly
Drink adequate volumes of water
If diabetic, control your blood sugar
Do not douche
If postmenopause, use vaginal oestrogen if not contraindicated
Sexual changes advised
Void after sex
Avoid anal intercourse (especially if followed by vaginal penetration)
Wash hands before sex
Drink water after sex
Wash genitals before and after sex
Use lubrication
If using sex toys ensure these are cleaned appropriately, regularly and stored properly

6.12   Conclusion

Recurrent urinary tract infections are a significant burden to the population of sexually active women and a cause of sexual avoidance or dysfunction for others. They can have debilitating effects on quality of life. It is known that sexual practices can exacerbate frequency of infections and thus reduce quality of life. Patients suffering from rUTI may avoid intercourse to prevent UTI. Even if intercourse is not avoided, hygiene measures to reduce risk of bacterial transmission may present a limitation for the sexual behaviour of some patients causing a detrimental effect on sexual function.

Clinicians should be aware of the close association between rUTI and sexual function. Efforts should be made to take an accurate history including sexual behavioural and hygiene practices and the temporal relationship of UTI to intercourse. Behavioural and hygiene advice should be given but we should be mindful that little of this is supported by evidence and that it may have a detrimental effect on the sexual function of these women.

References

Al Demour S, Ababneh MA (2018) Evaluation of behavioral and susceptibility patterns in pre-menopausal women with recurrent urinary tract infections: a case control study. Urol Int 100(1):31–36

Alós JI (2005) [Epidemiology and etiology of urinary tract infections in the community. Antimicrobial susceptibility of the main pathogens and clinical significance of resistance]. Enferm Infecc Microbiol Clin 23(suppl 4):3–8

Aydin A, Ahmed K, Zaman I, Khan MS, Dasgupta P (2015) Recurrent urinary tract infections in women. Int Urogynecol J 26(6):795–804

Bent S, Nallamothu BK, Simel DL, Fihn SD, Saint S (2002) Does this woman have an acute uncomplicated urinary tract infection? JAMA 287(20):2701–2710

Car J (2006) Urinary tract infections in women: diagnosis and management in primary care. BMJ 332(7533):94–97

Carlsen S, Krall SP, Xu KT, Tomanec A, Farias D, Richman P (2019) Sensitivity of urinary pathogens for patients discharged from the emergency department compared with the hospital anti-biogram. BMC Emerg Med 19(1):50

Cass AS, Ireland GW (1985) Antibacterial perineal washing for prevention of recurrent urinary tract infections. Urology 25(5):492–494

Christiaens TC, De Meyere M, Verschraegen G, Peersman W, Heytens S, De Maeseneer JM (2002) Randomised controlled trial of nitrofurantoin versus placebo in the treatment of uncomplicated urinary tract infection in adult women. Br J Gen Pract 52(482):729–734

Constantine ML, Pauls RN, Rogers RR, Rockwood TH (2017) Validation of a single summary score for the prolapse/incontinence sexual questionnaire-IUGA revised (PISQ-IR). Int Urogynecol J 28(12):1901–1907

Crann SE, Cunningham S, Albert A, Money DM, O'Doherty KC (2018) Vaginal health and hygiene practices and product use in Canada: a national cross-sectional survey. BMC Womens Health 18(1):52

Ejrnæs K (2011) Bacterial characteristics of importance for recurrent urinary tract infections caused by *Escherichia coli*. Dan Med Bull 58(4):B4187

Ellis AK, Verma S (2000) Quality of life in women with urinary tract infections: is benign disease a misnomer? J Am Board Fam Pract 13(6):392–397

Ennis SS, Guo H, Raman L, Tambyah PA, Chen SL, Tiong HY (2018) Premenopausal women with recurrent urinary tract infections have lower quality of life. Int J Urol 25(7):684–689

Excellence NIfHaC (2018) Urinary tract infection (lower):antimicrobial prescribing. NICE guideline [NG109]

Flores-Mireles AL, Walker JN, Caparon M, Hultgren SJ (2015) Urinary tract infections: epidemiology, mechanisms of infection and treatment options. Nat Rev Microbiol 13(5):269–284

Foxman B (1990) Recurring urinary tract infection: incidence and risk factors. Am J Public Health 80(3):331–333

Foxman B (2003) Epidemiology of urinary tract infections: incidence, morbidity, and economic costs. Dis Mon 49(2):53–70

Foxman B (2010) The epidemiology of urinary tract infection. Nat Rev Urol 7(12):653–660

Gardner A, Mitchell B, Beckingham W, Fasugba O (2014) A point prevalence cross-sectional study of healthcare-associated urinary tract infections in six Australian hospitals. BMJ Open 4(7):e005099

Heytens S, De Sutter A, Coorevits L, Cools P, Boelens J, Van Simaey L et al (2017) Women with symptoms of a urinary tract infection but a negative urine culture: PCR-based quantification of *Escherichia coli* suggests infection in most cases. Clin Microbiol Infect 23(9):647–652

Hooton TM (2001) Recurrent urinary tract infection in women. Int J Antimicrob Agents 17(4):259–268

Ikäheimo R, Siitonen A, Heiskanen T, Kärkkäinen U, Kuosmanen P, Lipponen P et al (1996) Recurrence of urinary tract infection in a primary care setting: analysis of a 1-year follow-up of 179 women. Clin Infect Dis 22(1):91–99

Kodner CM, Thomas Gupton EK (2010) Recurrent urinary tract infections in women: diagnosis and management. Am Fam Physician 82(6):638–643

Kornfält Isberg H, Melander E, Hedin K, Mölstad S, Beckman A (2019) Uncomplicated urinary tract infections in Swedish primary care; etiology, resistance and treatment. BMC Infect Dis 19(1):155

Kupelian AS, Horsley H, Khasriya R, Amussah RT, Badiani R, Courtney AM et al (2013) Discrediting microscopic pyuria and leucocyte esterase as diagnostic surrogates for infection in patients with lower urinary tract symptoms: results from a clinical and laboratory evaluation. BJU Int 112(2):231–238

Latthe PM, Toozs-Hobson P, Gray J (2008) Mycoplasma and ureaplasma colonisation in women with lower urinary tract symptoms. J Obstet Gynaecol 28(5):519–521

Lee BS, Bhuta T, Simpson JM, Craig JC (2012) Methenamine hippurate for preventing urinary tract infections. Cochrane Database Syst Rev 10:CD003265

Linder BJ, Bass EJ, Mostafid H, Boorjian SA (2018) Guideline of guidelines: asymptomatic microscopic haematuria. BJU Int 121(2):176–183

Malcolm W, Fletcher E, Kavanagh K, Deshpande A, Wiuff C, Marwick C et al (2018) Risk factors for resistance and MDR in community urine isolates: population-level analysis using the NHS Scotland Infection Intelligence Platform. J Antimicrob Chemother 73(1):223–230

Masajtis-Zagajewska A, Nowicki M (2017) New markers of urinary tract infection. Clin Chim Acta 471:286–291

Medina M, Castillo-Pino E (2019) An introduction to the epidemiology and burden of urinary tract infections. Ther Adv Urol 11:1756287219832172

Mercer CH, Tanton C, Prah P, Erens B, Sonnenberg P, Clifton S et al (2013) Changes in sexual attitudes and lifestyles in Britain through the life course and over time: findings from the National Surveys of Sexual Attitudes and Lifestyles (Natsal). Lancet 382(9907):1781–1794

Moskowitz D, Lee U (2018) Patient distress in women with recurrent urinary tract infections: how can physicians better meet patients needs? Curr Urol Rep 19(12):97

Naber KG, Bergman B, Bishop MC, Bjerklund-Johansen TE, Botto H, Lobel B et al (2001) EAU guidelines for the management of urinary and male genital tract infections. Urinary Tract Infection (UTI) Working Group of the Health Care Office (HCO) of the European Association of Urology (EAU). Eur Urol 40(5):576–588

Najeeb S, Munir T, Rehman S, Hafiz A, Gilani M, Latif M (2015) Comparison of urine dipstick test with conventional urine culture in diagnosis of urinary tract infection. J Coll Physicians Surg Pak 25(2):108–110

Nicolle LE, Ronald AR (1987) Recurrent urinary tract infection in adult women: diagnosis and treatment. Infect Dis Clin N Am 1(4):793–806

Nielsen AF, Walter S (1994) Epidemiology of infrequent voiding and associated symptoms. Scand J Urol Nephrol Suppl 157:49–53

Perrotta C, Aznar M, Mejia R, Albert X, Ng CW (2008) Oestrogens for preventing recurrent urinary tract infection in postmenopausal women. Cochrane Database Syst Rev (2):CD005131

Popkin BM, D'Anci KE, Rosenberg IH (2010) Water, hydration, and health. Nutr Rev 68(8):439–458

Renard J, Ballarini S, Mascarenhas T, Zahran M, Quimper E, Choucair J et al (2014) Recurrent lower urinary tract infections have a detrimental effect on patient quality of life: a prospective, observational study. Infect Dis Ther 4(1):125–135

Sahoo KC, Tamhankar AJ, Sahoo S, Sahu PS, Klintz SR, Lundborg CS (2012) Geographical variation in antibiotic-resistant *Escherichia coli* isolates from stool, cow-dung and drinking water. Int J Environ Res Public Health 9(3):746–759

Schmiemann G, Kniehl E, Gebhardt K, Matejczyk MM, Hummers-Pradier E (2010) The diagnosis of urinary tract infection: a systematic review. Dtsch Arztebl Int 107(21):361–367

Scholes D, Hooton TM, Roberts PL, Stapleton AE, Gupta K, Stamm WE (2000) Risk factors for recurrent urinary tract infection in young women. J Infect Dis 182(4):1177–1182

Schwenger EM, Tejani AM, Loewen PS (2015) Probiotics for preventing urinary tract infections in adults and children. Cochrane Database Syst Rev (12):CD008772

Stamey TA, Sexton CC (1975) The role of vaginal colonization with enterobacteriaceae in recurrent urinary infections. J Urol 113(2):214–217

Stamm WE, Counts GW, Running KR, Fihn S, Turck M, Holmes KK (1982) Diagnosis of coliform infection in acutely dysuric women. N Engl J Med 307(8):463–468

Su SB, Wang JN, Lu CW, Wang HY, Guo HR (2009) Prevalence of urinary tract infections and associated factors among pregnant workers in the electronics industry. Int Urogynecol J Pelvic Floor Dysfunct 20(8):939–945

Tanaka Y (2008) Immunosuppressive mechanisms in diabetes mellitus. Nihon Rinsho 66(12):2233–2237

Tandogdu Z, Wagenlehner FM (2016) Global epidemiology of urinary tract infections. Curr Opin Infect Dis 29(1):73–79

Wagenlehner F, Wullt B, Ballarini S, Zingg D, Naber KG (2018) Social and economic burden of recurrent urinary tract infections and quality of life: a patient web-based study (GESPRIT). Expert Rev Pharmacoecon Outcomes Res 18(1):107–117

Warren JW, Abrutyn E, Hebel JR, Johnson JR, Schaeffer AJ, Stamm WE (1999) Guidelines for antimicrobial treatment of uncomplicated acute bacterial cystitis and acute pyelonephritis in women. Infectious Diseases Society of America (IDSA). Clin Infect Dis 29(4):745–758

Yang B, Foley S (2018) First experience in the UK of treating women with recurrent urinary tract infections with the bacterial vaccine Uromune. BJU Int 121(2):289–292

Genitourinary Syndrome of Menopause and Female Sexual Dysfunction

Richard Flint and Cathy Davis

7.1 Introduction

Genitourinary syndrome of menopause (GSM) is the updated terminology of vulvo-vaginal atrophy (VVA) and was introduced in 2014 following a consensus statement from the International Society for the Study of Women's Health (ISSWH) and The North American Menopause Society (NAMS) (Portman et al. 2014). The GSM definition was introduced to describe more accurately the urogenital changes and the local symptoms occurring after the menopause in comparison to the terms of VVA/atrophic vaginitis. Hence, it involves clinical symptoms and signs from both the genital and the lower urinary tract (LUT) associated with the decreased hormone levels that can involve the labia majora/minora, vestibule/introitus, clitoris, vagina, urethra and bladder (Portman et al. 2014).

GSM affects up to 50% of postmenopausal women and 70% of breast cancer survivors (Mac Bride et al. 2010; Parish et al. 2013; The North American Menopause Society 2013), with women spending 40% of their lives postmenopausal. It is a chronic and progressive condition which unless treated is unlikely to improve over time and can have significant health sequela. GSM symptoms may also be mirrored in hypoestrogenic premenopausal women, these include women who are postnatal and exclusively breastfeeding, therefore not having periods and so not ovulating and those who are being treated for specific cancers such as breast cancer, with aromatase inhibitors (e.g. letrozole) or selective oestrogen receptor modulators (e.g. tamoxifen). GSM or its features manifests in 15% of premenopausal women (Palacios 2009).

GSM therefore is a common condition warranting close attention from healthcare providers, and public awareness on the topic should be increased. It is projected there will be more than 889 million women worldwide between the ages of 50 and

R. Flint (✉) · C. Davis
Urogynaecology Department, King's College Hospital, London, UK
e-mail: Richard.flint@nhs.net; cathydavis@nhs.net

© Springer Nature Switzerland AG 2021
A. Rantell (ed.), *Sexual Function and Pelvic Floor Dysfunction*,
https://doi.org/10.1007/978-3-030-63843-6_7

80 by 2020 and up to one-half of them will experience GSM symptoms at some point (DiBonaventura et al. 2015; Simon et al. 2018; Barlow et al. 1997a, b).

7.2   Signs and Symptoms

Although women may present with some or all of the clinical symptoms and signs, the most common symptom of VVA/GSM is vaginal dryness. Vaginal dryness appears at or soon after the menopause with a subsequent increase of prevalence as postmenopausal years' progress and is associated with an increase of LUTS. A longitudinal study of 438 women in Australia showed the prevalence of vaginal dryness increased with menopausal stage. Perimenopausal women had a prevalence of vaginal dryness of 4%, increasing to 25% at 1 year after the menopause and 47% at 3 years postmenopause (Dennerstein et al. 2000). It has been stated to be as high as 75% in the postmenopausal group (Gandhi et al. 2016). Other vaginal symptoms associated with GSM include vaginal burning, irritation and itching at the introitus. Such symptoms are often related to coital discomfort and pain with a consequent negative influence on female sexual function (Avis et al. 2018; Nappi et al. 2007).

Sexual function symptoms are also present with lack of lubrication, discomfort or pain during sexual intercourse and impaired sexual function. LUT symptoms of frequency, urgency, dysuria and recurrent urinary tract infections have also widely been reported. Symptoms are bothersome, cause personal distress and reduce quality of life (QOL) (DiBonaventura et al. 2015; Simon et al. 2013). The QOL impact of GSM is comparable with such serious medical conditions as arthritis, chronic obstructive pulmonary disease, asthma and irritable bowel syndrome (DiBonaventura et al. 2015).

Signs of GSM can include fissures at the posterior fourchette (small cuts/abrasions), labial resorption (where the labia minora, the smaller inner vulval lip becomes stuck to the outer lips and gradually regresses or is absorbed), pallor/erythema (pallor or redness to the area), loss of vaginal rugae (loss of folds of the vaginal tissue), protrusion of the urethral meatus (where the urethral opening becomes more prominent), urethral caruncle (benign fleshy outgrowth of the posterior urethral meatus), urethral prolapse/polyps and urethral sensitivity (Gandhi et al. 2016; Johnston et al. 2004). Other findings can include evidence of thinning or absent pubic hair, diminished elasticity and turgor of the vulvar skin and introital narrowing (Johnston et al. 2004; Nilsson et al. 1995). A detailed table of signs, symptoms and complications is shown in Table 7.1.

7.3   Diagnosis

GSM is primarily a clinical diagnosis based upon a patient's history and physical examination. Signs of GSM are noted in the previous section. It is important to add that only a weak correlation has been found between symptom score and physical examination of GSM (Davila et al. 2003). Objective tests of GSM include vaginal

Table 7.1 External genital, urological and sexual manifestations of genitourinary syndrome of menopause (Gandhi et al. 2016)

External genital		Urological		Sexual
Signs and symptoms	Complications	Signs and symptoms	Complications	Signs and symptoms
• Vaginal/pelvic pain and pressure • Dryness • Irritation/burning • Tenderness • Pruritus vulvae • Decreased turgor and elasticity • Suprapubic pain • Leukorrhea • Ecchymosis • Erythema • Thinning/greying pubic hair • Thinning/pallor of vaginal epithelium • Pale vaginal mucous membrane • Fusion of labia minora • Labial shrinking • Leukoplakic patches on vaginal mucosa • Presence of petechiae • Fewer vaginal rugae • Increased vaginal friability	• Labial atrophy • Vulvar atrophy and lesions • Atrophy of Bartholin glands • Intravaginal retraction of urethra • Alkaline pH (Gandhi et al. 2016) (5–7) • Reduced vaginal and cervical secretions • Pelvic organ prolapse • Vaginal vault prolapse • Vaginal stenosis and shortening • Introital stenosis	• Frequency • Urgency • Postvoid dribbling • Nocturia • Stress/urgency • Incontinence • Dysuria • Haematuria • Recurrent urinary tract infection	• Ischemia of vesical trigone • Meatal stenosis • Cystocele and rectocele • Urethral prolapse • Urethral atrophy • Retraction of urethral meatus inside vagina associated with vaginal voiding • Uterine prolapse • Urethral polyp or caruncle	• Loss of libido • Loss of arousal • Lack of lubrication • Dyspareunia • Dysorgasmia • Pelvic pain • Bleeding or spotting during intercourse

pH, Vaginal Maturation Value (VMV) and the Vaginal Health Index Score (VHIS). VMV and VHIS will be explained in more detail later in this chapter.

A full history should initially be undertaken however paying close attention to any substances which are being used on the area directly or indirectly such as lubricants, soaps, spermicides, pantyliners, all of these may contain irritants (Gandhi et al. 2016). A drug and medical history should be taken as these may highlight possible causes or risk factors for GSM. Please see Table 7.2 for a list of known GSM risk factors.

When examining the patient with GSM, it may be necessary to use a smaller speculum due to possible introital narrowing, vaginal shortening and lack of elasticity of the vagina. Table 7.1 outlines the signs which may be found on pelvic examination.

The use of a speculum will allow you to obtain the pH of the vagina using sensitive and narrow pH window litmus paper at the vaginal vault. A measurement of 3.5–5 indicates a healthy vagina. Values higher than this denote GSM due to the change in vaginal microbiome becoming more alkaline (Nilsson et al. 1995). The premenopausal vaginal microbiome is made up of many different bacteria but mainly lactobacilli which gives an acidic pH. This changes to a more mixed germ flora with a pH of 6–7 as menopause ensues. Changes to the pH of the vagina make it more suspectable to pathological organisms which can increase both vaginal and urinary tract infections. Reference ranges of a pH of 5–5.49 could be indicative of mild atrophy, a pH of 5.5–6.49 could be indicative of moderate atrophy, and a pH higher than 6.5 could be indicative of severe atrophy (Weber et al. 2015).

The VMV is an objective way of determining the degree of vaginal atrophy. To calculate the VMV, a smear is taken by scraping the upper third of the vaginal wall with a spatula. Samples are then transferred to a microscope slide, fixed and examined. The VMV or Vaginal Maturation Value quantifies the different layers of the vaginal epithelium by comparing percentages of parabasal, intermediate and superficial cells in a lab setting. The index is read from left to right, for example, a VMI of 0/30/70 represents 0% parabasal cells, 30% intermediate cells and 70% superficial cells. A shift to the left indicates an increase in the parabasal or intermediate

Table 7.2 Risk factors for GSM (Gandhi et al. 2016)

Risk factors for genitourinary syndrome of menopause
Menopause
Nonmenopause hypoestrogenism
Bilateral oophorectomy
Cigarette smoking
Alcohol abuse
Decreased frequency and sexual abstinence
Ovarian failure
Lack of exercise
Absence of vaginal childbirth

cells, while a shift to the right reflects an increase in the superficial or intermediate cells. A lower value indicates fewer superficial cells which is indicative of absent or very low oestrogen levels (Weber et al. 2015).

The Vaginal Health Index Score (VHIS) is a semi objective way of quantifying vaginal atrophy, it includes scoring of vaginal moisture, vaginal fluid volume, vaginal elasticity, vaginal pH and vaginal epithelial integrity on a scale of 1 (poorest) to 5 (best). The lower the score, the greater the atrophy (Bachmann 1994). Vaginal moisture is an assessment of the appearance and spread or consistency of the secretions which coat the vagina. Vaginal elasticity is a measure of the ability of the vaginal tissue to stretch from the examiner's finger. Vaginal epithelial integrity takes into account colour, thickness and ability of the tissue to resist breaking secondary to touch (Manonai et al. 2006). The only objective measure is pH, with the other four variables allowing an element of subjectivity. For that reason, no reproducibility studies have been published. Figure 7.1 shows the VHIS.

Score	1	2	3	4	5
Elasticity	None ☐	Poor ☐	Fair ☐	Good ☐	Excellent ☐
Fluid Volume (Pooling of secretion)	None ☐	Scant ☐ amount, vault not entirely covered	Superficial ☐ amount of dryness (small areas of dryness on cotton tip applicator)	Moderate ☐ amount of dryness (small areas of dryness on cotton tip applicator)	Normal ☐ amount (fully saturates on cotton tip applicator)
Ph (please also write the exact (or closest to the exact) value of pH as it is observed on the strip)	≥ 6.1 ☐	5.6 - 6.0 ☐	5.1 - 5.5 ☐	4.7 - 5.0 ☐	≤ 4.6 ☐ ....
Epithelial Integrity	Petechiae ☐ noted before contact	Bleeds ☐ with light contact	Bleeds ☐ with scraping	Not friable ☐ thin epithelium	Normal ☐
Moisture (Coating)	None ☐ surface inflamed	None ☐ surface not inflamed	Minimal ☐	Moderate ☐	Normal ☐

Fig. 7.1 VHIS

7.3.1   Physiological Changes

Anatomical and physiological changes which occur in the vagina and LUT during menopause are a direct consequence of reduced circulating oestrogen levels and the aging process (Mac Bride et al. 2010; Gandhi et al. 2016; Tan et al. 2012; Nappi and Palacios 2014). We know that the urethra and the bladder trigone originate embryologically from the same oestrogen receptor dense primitive urogenital sinus tissue, as are the vulvar vestibule and the upper vagina (Robinson et al. 2013). These oestrogen receptors in the vagina, vestibule and trigone of the bladder affect cellular proliferation and maturation and are important in the functioning of these organs (Mac Bride et al. 2010; Gandhi et al. 2016; Tan et al. 2012; Nappi and Palacios 2014). Therefore, reduced levels of circulating oestrogens both perimenopausal and postmenopausal result in changes to the urogenital tissues. During postmenopause, the number of receptors continue to decrease but do not disappear. Application of endogenous oestrogen replenishes these receptors allowing them to restore function (Palacios 2009; Gandhi et al. 2016). Failing that there is a reduction in collagen content and hyalinisation, decreased elastin, thinning of the epithelium and altered appearance and function of smooth muscle cells, increased density of connective tissue and fewer blood vessels. There are changes which affect the vulva with the labia minora thinning and regressing, and the introitus retracting and hymenal carunculate becoming smaller with loss of elasticity. Changes to the LUT include the urethral meatus appearing more prominent relative to the introitus and becoming vulnerable to physical irritation and trauma (Portman et al. 2014). Oestrogen is a vasoactive hormone that increases blood flow. Vaginal lubrication is caused by fluid transudation from blood vessels (fluid is pushed out of blood vessels into surrounding tissue to provide lubrication) and from the endocervical and Bartholin's glands. In the absence of oestrogen, this prolubricative function is lost. These physiological changes result in reduced vaginal blood flow, diminished lubrication, degreased flexibility and elasticity of the vaginal vault, shortening and narrowing of the vagina and increased vaginal pH (Mac Bride et al. 2010; Tan et al. 2012; Nappi and Palacios 2014). There is decreased vaginal tissue strength and increased friability which may predispose to epithelial damage with vaginal penetrative sexual intercourse, leading to vaginal pain, burning, fissuring, irritation and bleeding after sex (Mac Bride et al. 2010; Kingsberg et al. 2009). Epithelial thinning with decreased glycogenated superficial cells leads to changes in vaginal flora and loss of lactobacilli, increased vaginal pH and a change in the microbiome (Mac Bride et al. 2010; Hummelen et al. 2011; Brotman et al. 2014). The acidity of the vagina provides natural protection against urinary tract infections and vaginitis, discouraging the growth of pathogenic bacteria and infection. Therefore as a consequence, there is an increase in urinary tract and vaginal infections following an overgrowth of gram-negative rod faecal flora, including group B streptococci, staphylococci coliforms and diphtheroids (The North American Menopause Society 2007; Willhite and O'Connell 2001). With an increase in pathological organisms within the vagina and an increase in the amount of infections suffered, patients may then require courses of antibiotics and antifungal treatments to treat the change in flora and its resultant infections.

The female body produces three forms of oestrogen, these are: oestradiol, oestrone and oestriol. Oestradiol is most abundant in the premenopausal women. In postmenopausal women, the predominant oestrogen becomes oestrone which is less potent and therefore worsens the sequalae of reduced circulating oestrogen (Utian 1989).

7.3.2   Patient Awareness and Understanding

Patient understanding of GSM is poor within the general population. In the Vaginal Health: Insights, Views and Attitudes (VIVA) study, 45% of postmenopausal women reported that they experienced vaginal symptoms but only 4% identified these as being symptoms of VVA related to menopause (Nappi and Kokot-Kierepa 2012).

Lack of patient understanding and knowledge is likely worsened by limited interest of their healthcare providers. In the Real Women's Views of Treatment Options for Menopausal Vaginal Changes (REVIVE) survey, postmenopausal women reported that only 19% of healthcare professionals addressed their sexual lives and only 13% specifically raised the issue of genitourinary symptoms, despite the fact that 40% of women expected their healthcare professional to initiate discussions related to menopausal symptoms (Nappi et al. 2016). Barriers to discussing GSM include negative societal attitudes towards women's sexuality at older ages especially if the healthcare provider is younger or male (Lindau et al. 2007; Gott and Hinchliff 2003).

7.3.3   GSM and Sexual Dysfunction

The prevalence of female sexual dysfunction increases with age with nearly three quarters of women older than 60 years reporting sexual inactivity, difficulty with intercourse or dyspareunia (Diokno et al. 1990). Following a large-scale investigation of American women aged 18–102 years, we know the prevalence of any sexual problem was 44.2% (low desire, 38.7%; low arousal, 26.1% and orgasm difficulties, 20.5%), whereas sexually related personal distress was observed in only 22.8% of respondents. There was also a sharp age-dependent increase in the prevalence of all three sexual problems, with only 27.2% of women aged 18–44 years reporting any of the three problems, compared with 44.6% of middle-aged women (45–64 years) and 80.1% of elderly women (65 years or older) (Shifren et al. 2008).

When looking at GSM and sexual dysfunction, in the Menopause Epidemiology Study, 55% of sexually active women aged 40–65 years experienced female sexual dysfunction (FSD) and 57% VVA and those women with positive scores for FSD were almost four times more likely to have VVA as those women not reporting sexual symptoms (Levine et al. 2008). When looking at 1000 postmenopausal women and the effect VVA had on them, 64% reported painful sex, 64% described loss of libido and 58% admitted to avoiding intimacy (Simon et al. 2014). Other studies have reported that GSM impairs a women's level of sexual satisfaction (Kingsberg et al. 2013). This has led to a belief that the complex interaction of factors that affect sexual dysfunction in women after menopause might be associated with progressive vaginal atrophy (Nappi and Lachowsky 2009).

GSM has a significant impact on women's lives with one study reporting that 80% of women felt that VVA negatively impact their lives, particularly with regard to sensual intimacy (75%) and their ability to have a loving relationship (33%). Most (68%) felt that vaginal discomfort would make them feel less sexual. Almost 59% agreed (strongly or somewhat) that such symptoms could 'limit (their) comfort of doing what (they) want to do, when (they) want to do it, including sex', and 56% agreed that it could cause sexual problems with their partner (The North American Menopause Society 2013).

Sexual activity is already difficult to classify with a distinct lack of standardised terminology or definitions. However, if sexual activity is to include two persons (which strictly it does not), then it is reasonable to assume that in both hetero and homosexual relationships, with increasing age of one person, comes increasing age of the partner. In heterosexual relationships, with increasing male age comes increased prevalence of other medical comorbidities such as peripheral vascular disease, cardiac disease, diabetes, cancer, and prostate pathology, all of which impact on a male's sexual desire and ability to partake in sexual activity whether it be due to erectile dysfunction or changes in psychosexual thoughts and feelings, therefore will directly impact a female's sexual function if she depends on the male partner.

7.4 Treatment

The therapeutic management of GSM includes lubricants and moisturisers as first line therapy and low-dose vaginal oestrogens as second line, especially for women with a history of oestrogen dependent cancer. Oestrogen treatment is highly effective for GSM and related dyspareunia, being the most successful treatment modality to improve the VMV (The North American Menopause Society 2013). Local oestrogen is preferred if vaginal dryness is the primary concern, and systemic oestrogen if features of menopause such as hot flushes, mood changes and bone changes are bothersome or a factor (The North American Menopause Society 2013; Basson et al. 2010; Suckling et al. 2006).

7.4.1 Lubricants and Moisturisers

Lubricants and moisturisers are first line therapies for mild GSM; however can only be used for symptom relief and during sexual intercourse. They do not restore the local physiology and they are ineffective when LUTS are present. Hence, vaginal oestrogens remain the only local therapeutic option for the restoration of local physiology and management of VVA symptoms and LUTS. Lubricants and moisturisers have been discussed in more detail in Chap. 11.

7.4.2 Physiotherapy

Women with GSM and sexual pain may have dysfunctional pelvic floor muscles, which may become tense or tight as result of ongoing vaginal dryness and discomfort or pain with sexual activity (Rosenbaum 2010; Faubion and Rullo 2015). Women's health physiotherapists can often go through the use of devices such as vaginal dilators or small vibrators which can aid in restoring form and function to the vagina alone or in combination with hormonal treatments. This is discussed in more detail in Chap. 13.

7.4.3 Homeopathic and Lifestyle Modifications

Approximately 10% of women will want to or attempt to manage their condition with homeopathic remedies (Gandhi et al. 2016). Over the counter, remedies containing phytoestrogens (plant-based oestrogens, namely soy) are being sold and may have some benefit; however, there is a lack of evidence mainly due to the lack of standardised preparations and strengths. Women should be made aware that there is currently no proven remedy that exerts an effect on the vaginal epithelium and treatment of GSM (Willhite and O'Connell 2001).

Increased sexual activity is advised to maintain robust vaginal muscle condition. There is a positive link between sexual activity and maintenance of vaginal elasticity and pliability as well as lubricative response to sexual stimulation. Sexual intercourse improves blood circulation to the vagina, and seminal fluid contains sexual steroids, prostaglandins and essential fatty acids which maintain vaginal tissue. Vulvovaginal tissue stretching also helps to promote vaginal elasticity. Masturbation or the use of sexual devices are options for patients without partners (The North American Menopause Society 2013; Gandhi et al. 2016).

Other interventions which may help include stress reduction therapy and psychological counselling for women who have non-organic causes of vaginal dryness. Cessation of smoking can also help improve symptoms. Loose fitting, cotton clothing may also be of some benefit via improving air circulation and discouraging growth of microorganisms (Gandhi et al. 2016).

7.4.4 Oestrogen Therapy

Oestrogen therapy has been proven to be successful in rapidly restoring vaginal epithelium and associated vasculature, improving vaginal secretions, lowering vaginal pH to restore healthy vaginal flora, and alleviating the overall vulvovaginal symptoms (Palacios et al. 2015). Contraindication to oestrogen therapy includes known or suspected cases of breast cancer, oestrogen-dependant cancers, undiagnosed vaginal bleeding, history of thromboembolism, endometrial hyperplasia or cancer, hypertension, hyperlipidaemia, liver disease, hypersensitivity to the active compounds in oestrogen therapy, history of stroke, coronary heart disease, pregnancy, smoking in those >35 years old, migraines with aura and acute cholecystitis/cholangitis (Gandhi et al. 2016).

7.4.5 Local Oestrogen Therapy

Local oestrogen therapy includes: oestradiol, oestriol and conjugated equine oestrogens. Local therapy is the most acceptable form of therapy and offers the fastest and most effective symptomatic relief (Gandhi et al. 2016). Local oestrogen therapy is under prescribed despite being efficacious at treating GSM symptoms, with an Australian study reporting only 4.5% of women aged 40–65 years using vaginal oestrogen therapy (VET) (Worsley et al. 2016) and an American study showing 6% of women with a mean age of 58 years using VET. VET however also has a high discontinuation rate, with between 55% and 80% of women stopping treatment due to fears over adverse effects from use, lack of efficacy, cost or other reasons (Gandhi et al. 2016; Kyvernitakis et al. 2015a, b; Portman et al. 2015; Rahn et al. 2015). It is important to make patients aware that benefit will cease if the patient stops using the local oestrogen.

It is important to note that local oestrogen therapy has no effect on systemic menopausal symptoms of vasomotor hot flushes, bone mineral density loss, mood changes, etc. Common side effects include vaginal secretions, spotting and itching (Gandhi et al. 2016). As the local oestrogen only acts locally, there is limited systemic absorption by avoidance of hepatic metabolism. Therefore, progestogens are not required to prevent endometrial hyperplasia unlike with systemic oestrogen therapy. Local oestrogen therapy is for the alleviation of vaginal and LUT symptoms and their associated sexual dysfunction symptoms only (Gandhi et al. 2016).

With regard to route of administration, a 2006 Cochrane review found that all routes were equally as effective in alleviating symptoms of dyspareunia, dryness and itching (Suckling et al. 2006). Creams are currently the most popular choice of vaginal product as they provide flexibility of dosing and frequency of administration. Table 7.3 shows the available vaginal preparations. Women on local oestrogen therapy report 80–90% subjective improvement and relief from GSM (The North American Menopause Society 2013; Willhite and O'Connell 2001; Goldstein 2010). With regard to practicality, patient choice should take priority with respect to cream or pessary. The cream comes with an applicator which can be injected into the vagina; however, some patients may find this uncomfortable. Therefore, the same amount can be applied to a digit and can be manually inserted into the vagina which some patients find more acceptable. All pessaries are delivered via an applicator. Patients can experience a discharge as a result of the local oestrogen therapy and you may find that changing from one preparation to another may improve this.

Table 7.3 Preparations and strengths of vaginal oestrogen therapy

Product type	Generic name of active component	Brand name	Strength	Treatment
Vaginal cream	Oestriol	Gynest	0.01%	1× day for 2/52 then 2× week continuously
		Ovestin	0.1%	1× day for 3/52 then 3× week continuously
Vaginal pessary	Oestradiol	Vagifem	10 μg	1× day for 2/52 then every other day continuously
Vaginal ovule	Oestradiol	Imvexxy	4 μg 10μg	1× day for 2/52 then 2× week continuously
Vaginal ring	Oestradiol	Estring	7.5 μg/24 h	Replace every 90 days

7.4.6 Systemic Oestrogen Therapy

Both systemic and local oestrogen is effective; however, it is important to note that 40% of women on systemic oestrogen may still suffer GSM symptoms. The initiation of systemic oestrogen therapy should be weighed against the possible risks associated with its use and only commenced after a thorough review of the patient, taking into account their wishes also. If using, the lowest effective dose is advisable as the stimulatory effect of the oestrogen on the endometrium can lead to proliferation, hyperplasia or carcinoma (Gandhi et al. 2016). Systemic oestrogen should be reserved for those with other systemic menopausal symptoms such as hot flushes or osteoporosis (Brockie 2013).

Systemic oestrogen is also associated with breast tenderness and or enlargement, vaginal bleeding or spotting, nausea and modest weight gain. If a patch/transdermal approach is taken, then there can be irritant at the application sites. The most common side effect is increased systemic oestrogen which has risk associated with it as discussed before. Those women using systemic oestrogen who still have their uterus will need progestogen support to prevent the consequences of unopposed oestrogen, i.e. endometrial hyperplasia and eventual carcinoma. Those who have had a hysterectomy do not require progestogens. It is mainly the progestogens that increase the risk with this form of oestrogen therapy (Gandhi et al. 2016).

A Cochrane review showed that hormone therapy (oestrogen alone or in combination with a progestogen) was associated with a small to moderate improvement in sexual function, especially pain, in symptomatic or early menopausal women (Nastri et al. 2013).

7.4.7 Testosterone

Testosterone has been used in the management of postmenopausal women especially in treating decreased or loss of libido. Studies showing the use of subcutaneous testosterone have shown improved physiological and psychological symptoms of menopause, including improvements in vaginal atrophy and sexual dysfunction (Glaser et al. 2011; Lobo et al. 2003; Hubayter and Simon 2008) though these are scant.

Topical vaginal testosterone has also been used for the treatment of GSM and sexual function (Raghunandan et al. 2010; Witherby et al. 2011; Fernandes et al. 2014; Dahir and Travers-Gustafson 2014; Melisko et al. 2017; Apperloo et al. 2006). Results have shown a lowering of vaginal pH, increase the proportion of vaginal lactobacilli, improved VMV and sexual function and lessened dyspareunia. Most studies include a daily dosing regimen; however, when comparable results are being achieved with intermitted low dose VET and compliance is already an issue, it is difficult to see how vaginal testosterone therapy would be more appealing.

7.4.8 Ospemifene

Ospemifene (Osphena) is a selective oestrogen receptor modulator that has been shown to improve the vaginal maturation value, vaginal pH and symptoms of vaginal dryness (The North American Menopause Society 2013; Portman et al. 2013; Goldstein et al. 2014). It is an oral treatment option of 60 mg/day. Current literature shows, it is efficacious and safe in treating VVA and dyspareunia by improving vaginal structure and pH (Paton 2014). Trials showed that at 52 weeks there were no cases of endometrial cancer and <1% of patients suffered from endometrial hyperplasia. Contraindications include a history of thromboembolism. Common side effects reported by patients include a feeling of warmth/redness of the face, neck, arms, and occasionally, upper chest, sudden sweating and white or brownish vaginal discharge.

7.4.9 Dehydroepiandrosterone (DHEA)

Intravaginal DHEA (Prasterone) has been approved by the US Food and Drug Administration for the management of moderate-to-severe dyspareunia due to menopause, though this is currently the only country to licence the product. It is hypothesised that intravaginal DHEA is converted to oestrogens and androgens (Witherby et al. 2011). A placebo-controlled trial of daily insertion of 0.5% DHEA decreased vaginal pH, improved the VMV and vaginal epithelial thickness and integrity and increased vaginal secretion resulting in improvement in dyspareunia and all domains of sexual function as assessed by the Female Sexual Function Index (FSFI) (Labrie et al. 2015); however, more research is needed.

It has been noted that application of DHEA vaginally to women with sexual dysfunction but without VVA has still led to an improvement in their sexual function. Therefore it has controversially been hypothesised whether VVA and sexual dysfunction are two separate medical entities which are independently controlled by the sex steroids made locally in the vagina from the precursor DHEA of either endogenous or exogenous origin (Labrie et al. 2015).

Prasterone (Intrarosa) has now been approved on many UK hospital formularies. Current dosing regimen of prasterone is via 6.5 mg pessary, one pessary once a day, at bedtime. This can be inserted into the vagina with your finger or with an applicator provided in the pack. The most common side effect reported is vaginal discharge.

7.4.10 Vaginal Laser

Vaginal laser is novel treatment of GSM. Laser has been proven to be beneficial in treating GSM (Pitsouni et al. 2017), and as efficacious as standard therapy with local vaginal oestrogen. There are currently two main types of laser on the market, these are the microablative fractional CO_2 laser (SmartXide2 V2LR, Monalisa Touch, DEKA, Florence, Italy) and Non-ablative photothermal Erbium:YAG laser (Er:YAG-laser) (FotonaSmooth™ XS, Fotona, Ljubljana Slovenia). Both lasers ultimately cause thermomodulation by heating and (in the case of the CO_2) ablating columns of tissue. This leads to a controlled temperature rise, which in turn causes vasodilatation, collagen remodelling, collagen synthesis, neo-vascularisation and elastin formation, resulting in improved vaginal tissue tightness and elasticity and restoring vaginal flora to premenopausal status with predominant lactobacilli. Initial treatment is with between 3 and 5 sessions of laser, 4 weeks apart followed by a 'top up' once every year. There are currently no data over which laser is more beneficial to patients; however, research is currently being undertaken in this area (Flint et al. 2019).

Specific research into the use of vaginal laser and sexual function as well as GSM has been undertaken. A review of the literature showed that compared with baseline, following application of vaginal laser, dyspareunia significantly decreased in severity and the patient's perception of overall sexual function showed a significant improvement in each domain of the FSFI at last follow up (Salvatore et al. 2017).

7.4.11 MDT

An MDT approach should be taken with these patients as the disease can often be multifactorial. Patients may often present with GSM but may also suffer urinary incontinence, pelvic organ prolapse or bowel problems. Having a multidisciplinary service of doctors, nurse specialist, physiotherapists, vulval experts, dermatologists will lead to more joined up thinking and holistic care of the patient and ultimately better management of the patient and improved patient satisfaction.

7.4.12 Differential Diagnosis of GSM

GSM may have significant overlap between other medical conditions. Differential diagnosis includes, bacterial vaginosis, trichomoniasis, candidiasis, contact irritants, foreign bodies and sexual trauma. Other diagnoses to consider include neoplasia and precancerous neoplasia of internal or external female genitalia, endocrine disorders, infections from body piercings, vaginal stenosis secondary to radiation, lichen sclerosus and lichen planus (Goldstein 2010). There should be a low threshold to refer these patients to a specialist vulval clinic if the diagnosis is uncertain or the patient is not responding to standard treatments as there could either be a missed diagnosis or dual pathology.

7.5 Conclusion

GSM has a significant impact on a women's health-related quality of life including sexual dysfunction. Close attention should be paid to asking patients about GSM symptoms and picking on signs during pelvic examination. Tools such as vaginal pH and the VHIS may be reproducible within the clinic setting.

There are good treatment modalities available for the treatment of GSM and any associated sexual dysfunction symptoms. Mainstay of treatment is with topical local oestrogen therapy; however, there are other efficacious options available. With improving vaginal atrophy comes improvement in associated sexual dysfunction.

Sexual dysfunction in this cohort can often be multifactorial however and so the holistic treatment of the patient is paramount.

References

Apperloo M ct al (2006) ENDOCRINOLOGY: vaginal application of testosterone: a study on pharmacokinetics and the sexual response in healthy volunteers. J Sex Med 3(3):541–549

Avis NE et al (2018) Correlates of sexual function among multi-ethnic middle-aged women: results from the Study of Women's Health Across the Nation (SWAN). Menopause 25(11):1244–1255

Bachmann G (1994) Vulvo-vaginal complaints. In: Lobo R (ed) Treatment of the postmenopausal woman. Elsevier, Amsterdam

Barlow D, Samsioe G, Van Geelen J (1997a) A study of European womens' experience of the problems of urogenital ageing and its management. Maturitas 27(3):239–247

Barlow DH et al (1997b) Urogenital ageing and its effect on sexual health in older British women. BJOG Int J Obstet Gynaecol 104(1):87–91

Basson R et al (2010) Summary of the recommendations on sexual dysfunctions in women. J Sex Med 7(1pt2):314–326

Brockie J (2013) Managing menopausal symptoms: hot flushes and night sweats. Nurs Stand 28(12):48–53

Brotman RM et al (2014) Association between the vaginal microbiota, menopause status and signs of vulvovaginal atrophy. Menopause (New York, NY) 21(5):450

Dahir M, Travers-Gustafson D (2014) Breast cancer, aromatase inhibitor therapy, and sexual functioning: a pilot study of the effects of vaginal testosterone therapy. Sex Med 2(1):8–15

Davila GW et al (2003) Are women with urogenital atrophy symptomatic? Am J Obstet Gynecol 188(2):382–388

Dennerstein L et al (2000) A prospective population-based study of menopausal symptoms. Obstet Gynecol 96(3):351–358

DiBonaventura M et al (2015) The association between vulvovaginal atrophy symptoms and quality of life among postmenopausal women in the United States and Western Europe. J Women's Health 24(9):713–722

Diokno AC, Brown MB, Herzog AR (1990) Sexual function in the elderly. Arch Intern Med 150(1):197–200

Faubion SS, Rullo JE (2015) Sexual dysfunction in women: a practical approach. Am Fam Physician 92(4):281–288

Fernandes T, Costa-Paiva LH, Pinto-Neto AM (2014) Efficacy of vaginally applied estrogen, testosterone, or polyacrylic acid on sexual function in postmenopausal women: a randomized controlled trial. J Sex Med 11(5):1262–1270

Flint R et al (2019) Rationale and design for fractional microablative CO2 laser versus photothermal non-ablative erbium: YAG laser for the management of genitourinary syndrome of menopause: a non-inferiority, single-blind randomized controlled trial. Climacteric 22(3):307–311

Gandhi J et al (2016) Genitourinary syndrome of menopause: an overview of clinical manifestations, pathophysiology, etiology, evaluation, and management. Am J Obstet Gynecol 215(6):704–711

Glaser R, York AE, Dimitrakakis C (2011) Beneficial effects of testosterone therapy in women measured by the validated Menopause Rating Scale (MRS). Maturitas 68(4):355–361

Goldstein I (2010) Recognizing and treating urogenital atrophy in postmenopausal women. J Women's Health 19(3):425–432

Goldstein S et al (2014) Ospemifene 12-month safety and efficacy in postmenopausal women with vulvar and vaginal atrophy. Climacteric 17(2):173–182

Gott M, Hinchliff S (2003) Barriers to seeking treatment for sexual problems in primary care: a qualitative study with older people. Fam Pract 20(6):690–695

Hubayter Z, Simon J (2008) Testosterone therapy for sexual dysfunction in postmenopausal women. Climacteric 11(3):181–191

Hummelen R et al (2011) Vaginal microbiome and epithelial gene array in post-menopausal women with moderate to severe dryness. PLoS One 6(11):e26602

Johnston SL et al (2004) The detection and management of vaginal atrophy. J Obstet Gynaecol Can 26(5):503–515

Kingsberg S, Kellogg S, Krychman M (2009) Treating dyspareunia caused by vaginal atrophy: a review of treatment options using vaginal estrogen therapy. Int J Women's Health 1:105

Kingsberg SA et al (2013) Vulvar and vaginal atrophy in postmenopausal women: findings from the REVIVE (REal Women's VIews of Treatment Options for Menopausal Vaginal Chang Es) Survey. J Sex Med 10(7):1790–1799

Kyvernitakis I et al (2015a) Discontinuation rates of menopausal hormone therapy among postmenopausal women in the post-WHI study era. Climacteric 18(5):737–742

Kyvernitakis I et al (2015b) Persistency with estrogen replacement therapy among hysterectomized women after the Women's Health Initiative study. Climacteric 18(6):826–834

Labrie F et al (2015) Effect of intravaginal prasterone on sexual dysfunction in postmenopausal women with vulvovaginal atrophy. J Sex Med 12(12):2401–2412

Levine KB, Williams RE, Hartmann KE (2008) Vulvovaginal atrophy is strongly associated with female sexual dysfunction among sexually active postmenopausal women. Menopause 15(4):661–666

Lindau ST et al (2007) A study of sexuality and health among older adults in the United States. N Engl J Med 357(8):762–774

Lobo RA et al (2003) Comparative effects of oral esterified estrogens with and without methyltestosterone on endocrine profiles and dimensions of sexual function in postmenopausal women with hypoactive sexual desire. Fertil Steril 79(6):1341–1352

Mac Bride MB, Rhodes DJ, Shuster LT (2010) Vulvovaginal atrophy. In: Mayo clinic proceedings. Elsevier, Amsterdam

Manonai J et al (2006) The effect of a soy-rich diet on urogenital atrophy: a randomized, crossover trial. Maturitas 54(2):135–140

Melisko ME et al (2017) Vaginal testosterone cream vs estradiol vaginal ring for vaginal dryness or decreased libido in women receiving aromatase inhibitors for early-stage breast cancer: a randomized clinical trial. JAMA Oncol 3(3):313–319

Nappi R, Kokot-Kierepa M (2012) Vaginal health: insights, views & attitudes (VIVA)–results from an international survey. Climacteric 15(1):36–44

Nappi RE, Lachowsky M (2009) Menopause and sexuality: prevalence of symptoms and impact on quality of life. Maturitas 63(2):138–141

Nappi R, Palacios S (2014) Impact of vulvovaginal atrophy on sexual health and quality of life at postmenopause. Climacteric 17(1):3–9

Nappi R et al (2007) Aging and sexuality in women. Minerva Ginecol 59(3):287–298

Nappi RE et al (2016) The REVIVE (REal Women's VIews of Treatment Options for Menopausal Vaginal ChangEs) Survey in Europe: country-specific comparisons of postmenopausal women's perceptions, experiences and needs. Maturitas 91:81–90

Nastri CO et al (2013) Hormone therapy for sexual function in perimenopausal and postmenopausal women. Cochrane Database Syst Rev 6:CD009672

Nilsson K, Risberg B, Heimer G (1995) The vaginal epithelium in the postmenopause—cytology, histology and pH as methods of assessment. Maturitas 21(1):51–56

Palacios S (2009) Managing urogenital atrophy. Maturitas 63(4):315–318

Palacios S et al (2015) Update on management of genitourinary syndrome of menopause: a practical guide. Maturitas 82(3):308–313

Parish SJ et al (2013) Impact of vulvovaginal health on postmenopausal women: a review of surveys on symptoms of vulvovaginal atrophy. Int J Women's Health 5:437

Paton D (2014) Ospemifene for the treatment of dyspareunia in postmenopausal women. Drugs Today 50(5):357–364

Pitsouni E et al (2017) Laser therapy for the genitourinary syndrome of menopause. A systematic review and meta-analysis. Maturitas 103:78–88

Portman DJ et al (2013) Ospemifene, a novel selective estrogen receptor modulator for treating dyspareunia associated with postmenopausal vulvar and vaginal atrophy. Menopause 20(6):623–630

Portman DJ, Gass ML, Panel VATCC (2014) Genitourinary syndrome of menopause: new terminology for vulvovaginal atrophy from the International Society for the Study of Women's Sexual Health and the North American Menopause Society. Climacteric 17(5):557–563

Portman D et al (2015) One-year treatment persistence with local estrogen therapy in postmenopausal women diagnosed as having vaginal atrophy. Menopause 22(11):1197–1203

Raghunandan C et al (2010) ENDOCRINOLOGY: a comparative study of the effects of local estrogen with or without local testosterone on vulvovaginal and sexual dysfunction in postmenopausal women. J Sex Med 7(3):1284–1290

Rahn DD et al (2015) Vaginal estrogen use in postmenopausal women with pelvic floor disorders: systematic review and practice guidelines. Int Urogynecol J 26(1):3–13

Robinson D, Toozs-Hobson P, Cardozo L (2013) The effect of hormones on the lower urinary tract. Menopause Int 19(4):155–162

Rosenbaum TY (2010) Musculoskeletal pain and sexual function in women. J Sex Med 7(2):645–653

Salvatore S et al (2017) Sexual function in women suffering from genitourinary syndrome of menopause treated with fractionated CO2 laser. Sex Med Rev 5(4):486–494

Shifren JL et al (2008) Sexual problems and distress in United States women: prevalence and correlates. Obstet Gynecol 112(5):970–978

Simon JA et al (2013) Vaginal health in the United States: results from the Vaginal Health Insights, Views & Attitudes Survey. Menopause 20(10):1043–1048

Simon JA et al (2014) Clarifying Vaginal Atrophy's Impact on Sex and Relationships (CLOSER) survey: emotional and physical impact of vaginal discomfort on North American postmenopausal women and their partners. Menopause 21(2):137–142

Simon JA et al (2018) The role of androgens in the treatment of genitourinary syndrome of menopause (GSM): International Society for the Study of Women's Sexual Health (ISSWSH) expert consensus panel review. Menopause 25(7):837–847

The North American Menopause Society (2013) Management of symptomatic vulvovaginal atrophy: 2013 position statement of The North American Menopause Society. Menopause 20(9):888–902

Suckling JA et al (2006) Local oestrogen for vaginal atrophy in postmenopausal women. Cochrane Database Syst Rev 4:CD001500

Tan O, Bradshaw K, Carr BR (2012) Management of vulvovaginal atrophy-related sexual dysfunction in postmenopausal women: an up-to-date review. Menopause 19(1):109–117

The North American Menopause Society (2007) The role of local vaginal estrogen for treatment of vaginal atrophy in postmenopausal women: 2007 position statement of The North American Menopause Society. Menopause (New York, NY) 14(3 Pt 1):355

Utian WH (1989) Biosynthesis and physiologic effects of estrogen and pathophysiologic effects of estrogen deficiency: a review. Am J Obstet Gynecol 161(6):1828–1831

Weber M, Limpens J, Roovers J (2015) Assessment of vaginal atrophy: a review. Int Urogynecol J 26(1):15–28

Willhite LA, O'Connell MB (2001) Urogenital atrophy: prevention and treatment. Pharmacotherapy 21(4):464–480

Witherby S et al (2011) Topical testosterone for breast cancer patients with vaginal atrophy related to aromatase inhibitors: a phase I/II study. Oncologist 16(4):424–431

Worsley R et al (2016) Low use of effective and safe therapies for moderate to severe menopausal symptoms: a cross-sectional community study of Australian women. Menopause 23(1):11–17

Introducing the Subject to Women

Angie Rantell

8.1 Introduction

According to O'Donnell et al. (2005), only 24% of women were not at all embarrassed to discuss sexual problems with a healthcare professional (HCP) in comparison to 87% when discussing allergies or cold/flu. Approximately a third of women would not initiate a discussion about sexual issues with their doctors (Coyne et al. 2007). Rogers et al. (2018) report that many women are hesitant to initiate discussions on SF but want their HCP to open the dialogue. It is felt that by asking these questions, the HCP is acknowledging and prioritising the role that sexual health plays in overall well-being, and this will encourage the woman to openly discuss concerns so that an appropriate assessment can be performed. However, it has been shown that 74% of HCPs rely on their patients to initiate a discussion about sexual health (ARHP 2009).

This chapter aims to discuss how the topic of sexual activity (SA) and SF is introduced to women in the clinical setting. It will consider barriers to discussions, who's responsibility it is to initiate discussions and provide examples of conversation starters and screening questionnaires that can be used in practice.

8.2 Healthcare Professional Perspective

Communication between HCPs and patients about SF and pelvic floor dysfunction (PFD) has long been problematic, and there are still many clinicians who do not approach the topic of SF in patients with LUTD. Up to 60% of women attending urogynaecology clinics report sexual dysfunction (SD); however, only a minority are consistently screened for sexual complaints (Pauls et al. 2006). In a study of

A. Rantell (✉)
Urogynaecology Department, King's College Hospital, London, UK
e-mail: angela.rantell@nhs.net

© Springer Nature Switzerland AG 2021
A. Rantell (ed.), *Sexual Function and Pelvic Floor Dysfunction*,
https://doi.org/10.1007/978-3-030-63843-6_8

Table 8.1 Are we asking the right questions? (Sobecki et al. 2012)

Question	% Routinely asking
Assessing sexual activity	63
Sexual problems	40
Sexual satisfaction	28
Sexual orientation/identity	27
Pleasure from sexual activity	13.8

members of the Dutch Urology Association, 40.3% did not think that SD was routinely relevant to urological practice (Siddall 2010).

Sobecki et al. (2012) undertook a study amongst American obstetricians and gynaecologists to understand firstly if they were asking women about SA and SF, and secondly if they were asking the right questions to encompasses all aspects of sexual health. As displayed in Table 8.1, only 63% were routinely asking women if they are sexually active and only 40% ask if they are experiencing any sexual problems. It is also noted in the study that 25% of clinicians reported expressing disapproval over patient's reported sexual practices.

8.3 Barriers to Discussions

It has been suggested that concerns about time restraints, lack of effective treatments and embarrassment may prevent women initiating a discussion about sexual concerns with their doctors (Kingsberg 2006). There have also been several other barriers identified by patients that they consider impact upon their ability to talk about sex with a HCP and these are reported in Box 8.1.

Box 8.1 Barriers Identified as to Why Patients Do Not Want to Talk About Sex
- Practical barriers.
- Emotional avoidance.
- Shyness.
- Stigma.
- Normal with aging mentality.
- Partners.
- Religious/cultural beliefs.
- Subjective nature of issue.

The barriers identified by HCPs are considered common perceptions. Reasons for not discussing SF have been reported in the literature as 'not my responsibility', 'lack of knowledge and experience', 'embarrassment', 'lack of time', 'nothing can be done about it' (Stead et al. 2003; Gott et al. 2004; Brandenburg and Bitzer 2009; Macdowall et al. 2010).

Dyer and das Nair (2013) performed a systematic review of qualitative research over the previous 10 years to look for common themes as to why HCPs do not want to talk about sex with patients. The themes identified are reported in Box 8.2.

Box 8.2 Common Themes for Why HCPs Do Not Talk About Sex
- 'Open up a can of worms'
- Lack of time.
- Lack of resources.
- Lack of training.
- Concern about knowledge and ability.
- Worry will cause offence.
- Personal discomfort.
- Lack of awareness about sexual issues.
- Opposite gender/race/age concerns.

According to Nappi and Lachowsky (2009), giving women the opportunity to talk about sexual problems is a fundamental part of healthcare. For the clinicians who assert that they lack experience and are embarrassed, it has been shown that barriers to assessing SF are of less concern in those who perform such consultations daily or weekly compared to those who do so infrequently (Temple-Smith et al. 1999).

Currently in the UK and Europe, the most commonly used guidelines in the assessment of PFD are National Institute for Health and Care Excellence NG23 (NICE 2013), The International Consultation on Incontinence (ICI) recommendations (Abrams et al. 2017) and the EAU guideline on Urinary Incontinence (Nambiar et al. 2018), yet none of these mention questioning patients regarding SA as part of their routine assessment recommendations. The suggestion that assessment of SA should be incorporated into best practice standards/guidelines would help to start to break down these barriers and ensure that HCPs engage in these conversations more frequently which may help to normalise the issue.

8.4   Current Practice

In 2016, a survey was performed amongst an international group of clinicians treating men and women with lower urinary tract symptoms (LUTS) (Rantell et al. 2016). In this population, 71% of HCPs routinely ask patients with LUTS about SF and 86% of them feel comfortable doing so if the patient is heterosexual. If the patient was not sexually active (NSA), only 37% of clinicians probed further to understand why not, for example lack of partner or due to other health reasons.

When considering the specific aspects of SF for women, very few question about sexual satisfaction, arousal and ability or inability to achieve orgasm, instead focussing on pain or incontinence during sex. Almost 50% of HCPs did not

Table 8.2 Results of questionnaire related to female patients (Rantell et al. 2016)

Question	No of HCPs ($n = 35$)
Do you routinely ask patients with LUTS about SF?	71%
Do you feel comfortable asking about SF?	91%
If you know a person is sexually active do you routinely ask about	
(a) Satisfaction of sexual relationship	31%
(b) Arousal and lubrication	31%
(c) Ability to achieve orgasm	20%
(d) Pain during sex	83%
(e) Incontinence during sex or on orgasm	77%
(f) Worsening of urinary symptoms post intercourse	54%
(g) Comments/complaints from partner	20%
If a woman reports sexual dysfunction do you routinely ask about	
(a) Frequency of sexual activity	37%
(b) Severity of symptoms	74%
(c) Type of sexual activity	51% do not ask
	17% only vaginal
	9% all types (anal/oral/ masturbation)
(d) Bothersomeness	77%
(e) Psychological impact	49%
(f) If partner is aware	34%

question the type of SA a woman is practicing, with only 9% enquiring about all types of SA (vaginal/anal/oral/masturbation). Frequency of SA is rarely considered but if a woman reports some form of sexual dysfunction, the severity of symptoms and bothersomeness is regularly assessed. These results are displayed in full in Table 8.2.

8.5   What About Those Who Are Not Sexually Active (NSA)?

For many women, just because they are NSA at that time, they may not want the conversation to stop there. Women have reported feelings of exclusion and that they are missing something if not asked (Rantell 2019). Many may not be SA due to their PFD or other medical conditions whereas for others it may be due to partner issues or lack of a partner. For these women, it was highlighted that just because they are NSA at that time, does not mean that they are not seeking a relationship, and that in reality there are a whole different group of concerns and issues that women have in restarting, or seeking new sexual relationships. These may be related to body image/ desirability/performance and if there are additional concerns associated with LUTS, for example fear of leakage/smelling during sex or the concerns over disposal of incontinence pads, these increased anxieties may further restrict or prevent women from engaging in new sexual relationships (Rantell 2019). Further research into this concept is necessary to fully understand the issue and how HCPs may help and guide women to overcome this barrier.

For the clinicians who do not probe further regarding why a patient is NSA, they report it is either because they feel it is not relevant to the discussion or because of significant comorbidities that they think are likely to be the cause, for example mental health issues or neurological disability, or if patients expressed discomfort with the topic. Other reasons cited include the age and social status of the patient, if they were widowed, time constraints, forgetfulness (of the patient!) and if the patient was receiving treatment for cancer (Rantell et al. 2016).

Many of the reasons for not asking when someone is NSA actually go against the current literature. Studies have shown that up to 60% of older adults still want to be SA (Camacho and Reyes-Ortiz 2005) but are more likely to have sexual problems thus further probing in this group is essential (Laumann and Waite 2008). It has however been shown that it is the older adults who self-report good health who are more likely to be SA (Lindau et al. 2007). It has been suggested that the issue of sexuality, sexual health and older people appears to be another domain, which has been deeply infiltrated by ageism amongst HCPs (Bouman and Arcelus 2001; Weeks 2002) and embarrassment of the HCP when assessing sexual function has been cited as a causative factor (Bouman et al. 2006).

Medical comorbidities, for example diabetes and hypertension, are often the cause of sexual problems but this is not always the case and other underlying reversible problems should be ruled out. In line with this, current literature in diabetes management recommends that sexual health should be broadly assessed in both SA and sexually inactive people with type 2 diabetes (Bjerggaard et al. 2015). With regard to not asking patients with certain types and stages of cancer, evidence suggests that up to 74% of cancer patients and survivors thought that discussions with HCPs about sexual problems were important during and after treatment (Flynn et al. 2012).

8.6   Asking About Sexual Satisfaction/Frequency/ Partners Awareness

Sexual satisfaction is rarely questioned in practice. According to McClelland (2010), research on sexual satisfaction is in its infancy stage. A systematic review demonstrated the importance but also the complexity of sexual satisfaction and stated that there is a lack of theoretical models combining the most important aspects to explain sexual satisfaction (del Mar Sánchez-Fuentes et al. 2014). However, it is noted that there are many different facets to sexual satisfaction and this could potentially be why it is seldom questioned.

Frequency of sex is also rarely questioned according to this study, although the answer may help clinicians to gain a deeper insight into a person's sexual life and tailor appropriate therapy, for patients and their partners (del Mar Sánchez-Fuentes et al. 2014). However, the frequency of sex does not predict marital satisfaction (McNulty et al. 2016).

Very small numbers of HCPs ask patients if their partners are aware of the problem. In some cases, this may be obvious if the partner is present during the consultation; however, for others if there is poor communication amongst couples, this in itself can lead to reduced sexual satisfaction and impede intimacy. Research also suggests that a woman's sexual satisfaction predicts her partner's relationship satisfaction (Yoo et al. 2014).

8.7   LGBTQ+ Communities

It has long been noted that HCPs avoid discussions about same-sex orientations as a result of feeling uncomfortable talking about sex (Stein and Bonuck 2001). Research suggests that by trying to make improvements in communication about sexual health with lesbian and gay patients through training at undergraduate and postgraduate levels and by clinicians taking a proactive role during consultations, it may break down some of the barriers currently in place (Hinchliff et al. 2005). In the UK in 2017, NHS England released new guidelines, where HCPs in England are to be told to ask all patients aged 16 years or over about their sexual orientation, not only to gather data but also to ensure well-rounded healthcare services. By encouraging HCPs to broach the subject more frequently, it may help to reduce personal discomfort with the discussions (NHS England Equality and Health Inequalities Unit 2017).

Many HCPs may feel that they do not have the appropriate knowledge to be able to provide advice to this population of patients. However, the role of the HCP is not always to provide advice themselves but to signpost patients into the appropriate services, and there are now many that are specifically focused on the LGBTQ+ community. Therefore, HCPs should be educated to initiate the discussion and once a problem has been identified to have an awareness of local services available that they can refer the patient onto.

8.8   Presence of a Partner

Many clinicians felt the need to ask patients about SF when they are with a partner/relative and again when alone (Rantell 2019). This suggests the belief that patients do not always disclose all relevant information, especially if they do not want the person accompanying them to know that a problem exists or the extent of it or potentially just due to embarrassment. In general practice, HCPs have reported that people accompanying patients usually have a positive influence on medical encounters (Brown et al. 1998). However, this study included children and older adults attending GP surgeries for common medical conditions and not for problems associated with PFD and SF was unlikely to be relevant to many of these consultations. Partner communication appears to play an important role in both the quality of the marital relationship and degree of SD (McCabe and Cobain 1998). Witting et al. (2008) suggested that partner incompatibility was a factor in sexual dysfunction with specific complaints of 'too little foreplay' and 'partner more interested'. If a woman has not broached these issues with her partner at home, it raises the question of how likely she will be to mention it for the first time during a clinical consultation. Also, if the accompanying person is a family friend or advocate, many would not want him/her knowing their personal business. There is little in the literature about the impact of accompanying persons when a woman is undergoing a consultation regarding PFD and associated SF and there is also a lack of data regarding the partner response.

8.9   Who Should Ask the Questions?

Many HCPs feel that questions related to SF are better asked by someone of the same sex. Studies have shown that although many women (34–75%) do not have a preference for the sex of their gynaecologist (Fisher et al. 2002), for those who preferred a woman, it was quoted as due to either religious beliefs, the fact that a woman may understand their problems better and issues of personal modesty (Makam et al. 2010). A study interviewed male gynaecologists regarding discussing SF with women in clinical practice (Schweizer et al. 2013). One of the themes identified related to 'a sense of modesty' of their own as well as of their patients'. The analysis highlighted some fears, in male gynaecologists' discourses, of being perceived as intrusive by broaching the topic of sexuality.

Hall et al. (2002) performed a reciprocal likeability study and found that female clinicians like their patients more than male clinicians and that the patients liked their female clinicians more than the males. If a patient likes his/her HCP then this is going to help them feel more comfortable during personal discussions. Hojat (2007) reported that female clinicians score higher in empathy than their male counterparts and this was one of the important factors for women discussing SF. Interviews of women with LUTS regarding HCP–patient communication also found that women preferred to talk to a female HCP as many reported that their male clinician 'does not understand', 'is not concerned' or 'this is not important to him' and this led to an overall dissatisfaction with the quality of communication regarding OAB (Filipetto et al. 2014).

For some women, the age of the HCP that is asking the questions can be considered an issue. If the HCP was considered to be too young, it would change their initial preference in sex of the clinician. It has been reported that people stereotype on two different dimensions, the first being friend/foe (warmth) and the second being capability (competence) (Fiske et al. 1999). Whilst people stereotype their own preference as both warm and competent, they judge most outgroups ambivalently by ascribing both negative and positive characteristics to them. This is what appears to happen with sex and age of the clinician. Warm and competent is an older female clinician, warm but incompetent would be a young female clinician, cold but competent would be an old male clinician and the worst outcome of cold and incompetent is a young male clinician.

8.10   Timing of Discussions

There is no specific guidance as to when is the ideal point in a consultation for the discussion of SF to be initiated. Focus groups were held with women to understand how they want to be approached regarding SF (Rantell 2019). Some women feel that it is often asked as a final point towards the end of a discussion and that took away some of the importance of the discussion. They also felt that the clinicians did not really want to get into the discussion. Others are not concerned where in the conversation it took place as long as it happened. However, everyone was in agreement that it should not be at the beginning of a consultation, unless that was the presenting complaint. The length of time that people have for the discussion also raises concerns as it is not something that can be rushed and this does not always fit into short-time frames especially such as those in general practice clinics.

For nurses and AHPs, it is often common practice to meet the patients on several occasions over an extended period of time. This means that they ideally develop solid patient—clinician relationships which are a key feature to encouraging women to open up and feel comfortable discussing SF. As this group of clinicians often have longer appointments scheduled for these patients, it means that they are the ideal HCP to initiate and develop these discussions.

8.11   Initiating the Discussion: What Do Women Want?

There are many different views and variations on the way in which women have been approached about SF and very few studies investigating how they would have liked the topic to have been broached with them. Focus groups with women with PFD regarding discussing SF described three main areas for consideration (Rantell 2019).

1. A desire for prewarning.
2. Verbal questions/conversation starters related to how SF is introduced and how questions are asked.
3. Written methods of communication.

Most of the women agreed that one single method was not ideal and that using the written word as well as a conversation was the best approach (Rantell 2019).

8.12   Prewarning

It could be suggested that for women attending a clinic for PFD, it is not automatically considered by the patient that HCPs will be asking them about SF as they are concentrating on the presenting complaint. By having some idea before the clinic appointment about what to expect on the day and the sort of questions that may be asked, women feel that this would help them to mentally prepare for the appointment and consider if they wish to broach the subject of SF and what concerns they have (Rantell 2019).

The concept of prewarning about the context of consultations and the likelihood that intimate questions may be asked is not new. Tomlinson and Milgrom (1999) reported that some doctors get over their initial embarrassment and the shame/humiliation of the patient by giving them a preconsultation questionnaire that introduces the discussion and identifies concerns. However, this is not preferred by all, as many women dislike this anonymity and apparent coldness of this method. Although there are now many questionnaires to assess sexual function/sexual health and PFD in women, with a Grade A, B or C rating (Abrams et al. 2017), none of these contain questions relating to whether women wish to further discuss their concerns or answers on the questionnaire with their HCP. These questionnaires will be discussed in more depth in Chap. 10.

A more simple method of prewarning could be a simple change in the wording of the appointment letters that are sent to women. By adding an explanatory sentence that questions of an intimate/personal nature may be asked during the consultation, this would allow the patients to decide if they wish to bring a partner/friend into the consultation, or allow them to express a preference for the clinician that they see.

8.13 Verbal Communication/Conversation Starters

When discussing communication, it is not just the verbal but also the non-verbal cues that the patients pick up on. The tone of the questions is also important in helping the women feel at ease with discussions. The establishment of rapport within the consultation is a high priority for a lot of the women to feel that they could truly open up about their issues and associated feelings.

The way in which questions are phrased can significantly change the impact that they may have. By rephrasing questions to minimise impact and by ensuring that the woman understands why the clinician feels it is important to ask about SF, for example by linking it to common problems experienced by other women, it may normalise the issue, reduce embarrassment and help them to not feel alone. The aim of the conversation starter is not only to introduce the topic but also to gain initial consent to probe further. Using open rather than closed questions will help to develop a dialogue that will enable further assessment of SF.

Examples of conversation starters include:

- I am going to ask you a few questions about your sexual history. I ask these questions at least once a year of all my patients because they are very important for your overall health. Everything you tell me is confidential. Do you have any questions before we start?
- Many women with PFD report that it can cause problems with their sexual relationships—is this something that you have noticed or would like to discuss?

Once the conversation has been started and the patient has reported a problem or concern and a desire for help, more in-depth questions can be asked to understand the specifics of their problem and impact on quality of life. This is discussed further in Chaps. 9 and 10.

The National Coalition for Sexual Health in America has published a document entitled 'Sexual Health and your Patients: A Provider's Guide' (Altarum Institute 2019). It details the key points to ensuring a productive SH conversation as displayed in Box 8.3.

Box 8.3 Key Points to Ensuring a Productive Sexual Health Conversion
- Assess your own comfort discussing sex with various patient groups and identify any biases that you may have. If you are uncomfortable talking about sex and sexuality, your patient will be too.
- Make your patient feel comfortable and establish rapport before asking sensitive questions.
- Use neutral and inclusive terms (e.g., "partner") and pose your questions in a non-judgmental manner.
- Avoid making assumptions about your patient based on age, appearance, marital status, or any other factor. Unless you ask, you cannot know a person's sexual orientation, behaviors, or gender identity.
- Try not to react overtly, even if you feel uncomfortable or embarrassed. Pay attention to your body language and posture.
- Ask for preferred pronouns or terminology when talking to a transgender patient. Use those pronouns and support that patient's current gender identity, even if their anatomy does not match that identity.
- Rephrase your question or briefly explain why you are asking a question if a patient seems offended or reluctant to answer.
- Use ubiquity statements to normalize the topics you are discussing. These statements help patients understand that sexual concerns are common.
- Ensure that you and your patient share an understanding of the terms being used to avoid confusion. If you are not familiar with a term your patient used, ask for an explanation.

8.14   Role of Questionnaires

Questionnaires are used in many areas of clinical practice, and there are many to assess SF and its impact on QoL. However, one of the difficulties experienced is in making one tool relevant to all and with the topic of SF being so multifaceted, it raises the question if it will ever be possible to have a single tool that is suitable for all.

It has been acknowledged that for patients who find the discussion of intimate issues with HCPs very difficult, questionnaires may allow these issues to be measured in private, at ease and more effectively before exploring the questionnaire responses in a clinical interview (Abrams et al. 2017).

Questionnaires have also been developed to use as screening tools to identify women who report issues with SF and gain consent to further discuss the topic. The Brief Sexual Symptom Checklist for Women (BSSC-W) is a four-item questionnaire that assesses if a woman is SA, if they experience any problems with SA and if they would like to discuss this with a clinician. It was developed by the International Consultation in Sexual Medicine (ICSM) (Hatzichristou et al. 2004). The questionnaire is demonstrated in Fig. 8.1. Also available is the Sexual Complaints Screener for Women (SCS-W) which was developed by the Standards Committee of the International Society for Sexual Medicine and consists of a series of questions concerning sexual experiences during the last 6 months (Porst 2009). However, there are no validation studies available for these tools and there are no acknowledgements of PFD (Hatzichristou et al. 2010).

Brief Sexual Symptom Checklist for Women (BSSC-W)

Please answer the following questions about your overall sexual function

1. Are you satisfied with your sexual function?

☐ Yes   ☐ No

If No, please continue.

2. How long have you been dissatisfied with your sexual function?

....

3a. The problem(s) with your sexual function is: (mark one or more)

    1 Problem with little or no interest in sex

    2 Problem with decreased genital sensation (feeling)

    3 Problem with decreased vaginal lubrication (dryness)

    4 Problem reaching orgasm

    5 Problem with pain during sex

    6 Other:

3b. Which problem is most bothersome (circle)   1 2 3 4 5 6

4. Would you like to talk about it with your doctor?

☐ Yes   ☐ No

Fig. 8.1 Brief sexual symptom checklist for women (BSSC-W)

8.15 Healthcare Professional Education

HCP education relating to SF is lacking. In an ideal world, all HCPs would be provided with training to include ways in which to normalise the discussion about SF and appropriate language to use including how to individualise assessment and adapt their style of questioning and at what point in a clinical consultation these discussions are appropriate. Useful tools in practice including the use of diagrams to help explain conditions/problems to women should be made readily available. This training should also highlight that SA is a continuum and just because a woman may not be SA at one point of asking, it does not mean that is always going to be the case and that regular re-assessment in required. It is already routine practice to reassess SF in women post-surgery for PFD or post-partum, therefore this needs to extend to all women who are NSA attending our clinics and not just specific patient populations.

8.16 Conclusion

There are still many HCPs who do not approach the topic of SF in patients with PFD. For those who are, the majority are focussing on pain and symptoms during sex rather than understanding more about general sexual health, e.g. satisfaction and psychological impact or consider why women may not be sexually active. There are many perceived barriers to discussing SF; however, many of these can be overcome by HCP's being more open and asking the questions more frequently. Communication skills are paramount to facilitating discussion and no one approach is right for all so a combination of direct questioning and the use of standardised questionnaires should be considered. As sexual practices of patients are changing, HCP training in relation to SF in the LGBTQ+ community may need to be revised to ensure that this group of patients do not receive substandard care.

References

Abrams P, Cardozo L, Wein A, Wagg A (eds) (2017) Incontinence, 6th edn. Health Publications Ltd, Cork

Altarum Institute (2019) Sexual health and your patients: a providers guide. Altarum Institute, Washington, DC

ARHP. 2009. http://www.arhp.org/publications-and-resources/clinical-fact-sheets/shf-talking

Bjerggaard M, Charles M, Kristensen E, Lauritzen T, Sandbæk A, Giraldi A (2015) Prevalence of sexual concerns and sexual dysfunction among sexually active and inactive men and women with screen-detected type 2 diabetes. Sex Med 3:302–310

Bouman WP, Arcelus J (2001) Are psychiatrists guilty of ageism when it comes to taking a sexual history? Int J Geriatr Psychiatry 16:27–31

Bouman WP, Arcelus J, Benbow SM (2006) Nottingham study of sexuality & ageing (NoSSA I). Attitudes regarding sexuality and older people: a review of the literature. Sex Relatsh Ther 21(02):149–161

Brandenburg U, Bitzer J (2009) The challenge of talking about sex: the importance of patient–physician interaction. Maturitas 63(2):124–127

Brown JB, Brett P, Stewart M, Marshall JN (1998) Roles and influence of people who accompany patients on visits to the doctor. Can Fam Physician 44:1644

Camacho ME, Reyes-Ortiz CA (2005) Sexual dysfunction in the elderly: age or disease? Int J Impot Res 17:S52–S56

Coyne K, Margolis M, Jumadilova Z, Bavendeam T, Mueller E, Rogers R (2007) Overactive bladder and womens sexual health: what is the impact? J Sex Med 4(3):656–666

del Mar Sánchez-Fuentes M, Santos-Iglesias P, Sierra JC (2014) A systematic review of sexual satisfaction. Int J Clin Health Psychol 14(1):67–75

Dyer K, das Nair R (2013) Why don't healthcare professionals talk about sex? A systematic review of recent qualitative studies conducted in the United Kingdom. J Sex Med 10(11):2658–2670

NHS England Equality and Health Inequalities Unit (2017) Implementation guidance fundamental standard for sexual orientation monitoring. DOH, London

Filipetto FA, Fulda KG, Holthusen AE, McKeithen TM, McFadden P (2014) The patient perspective on overactive bladder: a mixed-methods needs assessment. BMC Fam Pract 15(1):96

Fisher WA, Bryan A, Devaitis KL, Silcox J, Kohn H (2002) It ain't necessarily so: most women do not strongly prefer female obstetrician-gynaecologists. J Obstet Gynaecol Can 24(11):885–888.

Fiske ST, Xu J, Cuddy AC, Glick P (1999) (Dis) respecting versus (dis) liking: status and interdependence predict ambivalent stereotypes of competence and warmth. J Soc Issues 55(3):473–489

Flynn KE, Reese JB, Jeffery DD, Abernethy AP, Lin L, Shelby RA, Porter LS, Dombeck CB, Weinfurt KP (2012) Patient experiences with communication about sex during and after treatment for cancer. Psycho-Oncology 21(6):594–601

Gott M, Galena E, Hinchliff S, Elford H (2004) "Opening a can of worms": GP and practice nurse barriers to talking about sexual health in primary care. Fam Pract 21(5):528–536

Hall JA, Horgan TG, Stein TS, Roter DL (2002) Liking in the physician–patient relationship. Patient Educ Couns 48:69–77

Hatzichristou D, Rosen RC, Broderick G, Clayton A, Cuzin B, Derogatis L, Litwin M, Meuleman E, O'leary M, Quirk F, Sadovsky R (2004) Clinical evaluation and management strategy for sexual dysfunction in men and women. J Sex Med 1(1):49–57

Hatzichristou D, Rosen RC, Derogatis LR, Low WY, Meuleman EJ, Sadovsky R, Symonds T (2010) Recommendations for the clinical evaluation of men and women with sexual dysfunction. J Sex Med 7(1pt2):337–348

Hinchliff S, Gott M, Galena E (2005) 'I daresay I might find it embarrassing': general practitioners' perspectives on discussing sexual health issues with lesbian and gay patients. Health Soc Care Community 13(4):345–353

Hojat M (2007) Empathy in patient care: antecedents, development, measurement, and outcomes. Springer, New York, NY

Ivins JP, Kent GG (1993) Women's preferences for male or female gynaecologists. J Reprod Infant Psychol 11(4):209–214

Kingsberg S (2006) Taking a sexual history. Obstet Gynaecol Clin North Am 6(33):535–547

Laumann EO, Waite LJ (2008) Sexual dysfunction among older adults: prevalence and risk factors from a nationally representative US probability sample of men and women 57–85 years of age. J Sex Med 5(10):2300–2311

Lindau ST, Schumm LP, Laumann EO, Levinson W, O'muircheartaigh CA, Waite LJ (2007) A study of sexuality and health among older adults in the United States. N Engl J Med 357(8):762–774

Macdowall W, Parker R, Nanchahal K, Ford C, Lowbury R, Robinson A, Sherrard J, Martins H, Fasey N, Wellings K (2010) 'Talking of sex': developing and piloting a sexual health communication tool for use in primary care. Patient Educ Couns 81(3):332–337

Makam A, Saroja CSM, Edwards G (2010) Do women seeking care from obstetrician–gynaecologists prefer to see a female or a male doctor? Arch Gynecol Obstet 281(3):443–447

McCabe MP, Cobain MJ (1998) The impact of individual and relationship factors on sexual dysfunction among males and females. Sex Marit Ther 13(2):131–143

McClelland SI (2010) Intimate justice: a critical analysis of sexual satisfaction. Soc Personal Psychol Compass 4(9):663–680

McNulty JK, Wenner CA, Fisher TD (2016) Longitudinal associations among relationship satisfaction, sexual satisfaction, and frequency of sex in early marriage. Arch Sex Behav 45(1):85–97

Nambiar AK, Bosch R, Cruz F, Lemack GE, Thiruchelvam N, Tubaro A, Bedretdinova DA, Ambühl D, Farag F, Lombardo R, Schneider MP (2018) EAU guidelines on assessment and nonsurgical management of urinary incontinence. Eur Urol 73(4):596–609

Nappi RE, Lachowsky M (2009) Menopause and sexuality: prevalence of symptoms and impact on quality of life. Maturitas 63(2):138–141

NICE (2013) CG171 female urinary incontinence. www.nice.org.uk

O'Donnell M, Lose G, Sykes D, Voss S, Hunskaar S (2005) Help seeking behaviour and associated factors amond women with urinary incontinence in France, Germany, Speain and the UK. Eur Urol 47:385–392

Pauls RN, Segal JL, Silva WA, Kleeman SD, Karram MM (2006) Sexual function in patients presenting to a urogynaecology practice. Int Urogynecol J Pelvic Floor Dysfunct 17(6):576–580

Porst H (2009) The Standards Committee of the International Society for Sexual Medicine the Sexual Complaints Screener for Men (SCS-M) and Women (SCS-W)

Rantell A (2019) How do women want to be approached about sexual function? In: AUGS/IUGA joint scientific meeting 2019. AUGS/IUGA

Rantell AM, Kelleher C, Cardozo L (2016) Sexual pursuits in clinical practice! Int Urogynecol J 27:S142–S143

Rogers RG, Pauls RN, Thakar R, Morin M, Kuhn A, Petri E, Fatton B, Whitmore K, Kingsberg SA, Lee J (2018) An international Urogynecological association (IUGA)/International Continence Society (ICS) joint report on the terminology for the assessment of sexual health of women with pelvic floor dysfunction. Int Urogynecol J 29(5):647–666

Schweizer A, Bruchez C, Santiago-Delefosse M (2013) Integrating sexuality into gynaecological consultations: gynaecologists' perspectives. Cult Health Sex 15(2):175–190

Siddall R (2010) Female sexual dysfunction: new developments. Trends Urol Gynaecol Sex Health 15(1):32–33

Sobecki JN, Curlin FA, Rasinski KA, Lindau ST (2012) What we don't talk about when we don't talk about sex: results of a national survey of US obstetrician/gynecologists. J Sex Med 9(5):1285–1294

Stead ML, Brown JM, Fallowfield L, Selby P (2003) Lack of communication between healthcare professionals and women with ovarian cancer about sexual issues. Br J Cancer 88(5):666–671

Stein GL, Bonuck KA (2001) Physician–patient relationships among the gay and lesbian community. J Gay Lesbian Med Assoc 5:87–93

Temple-Smith MJ, Mulvey G, Keogh L (1999) Attitudes to taking a sexual history in general practice in Victoria, Australia. Sex Transm Infect 75(1):41–44

Tomlinson J, Milgrom EC (1999) Taking a sexual history. West J Med 170(5):284

Weeks DJ (2002) Sex for the mature adult: health, self-esteem and countering ageist stereotypes. Sex Relatsh Ther 17(3):231–240

Witting K, Santtila P, Varjonen M, Jern P, Johansson A, Von Der Pahlen B, Sandnabba K (2008) Couples' sexual dysfunctions: female sexual dysfunction, sexual distress, and compatibility with partner. J Sex Med 5(11):2587–2599

Yoo H, Bartle-Haring S, Day RD, Gangamma R (2014) Couple communication, emotional and sexual intimacy, and relationship satisfaction. J Sex Marital Ther 40(4):275–293

9

Susan Kellogg Spadt and Lela Tannenbaum

9.1 Sexual Pain Disorders

Sexual pain is underreported by patients and often overlooked during office visits, as most providers do not ask directly about sexual function and dysfunction (Sorensen et al. 2018; Mitchell et al. 2017; Weiss et al. 2012). When women do complain of sexual pain, they often feel dismissed and invalidated, particularly if the aetiology is not easily identified (Sorensen et al. 2018). When addressed, it is often incorrectly diagnosed and poorly managed which can exacerbate patient distress.

Two terms commonly associated with chronic sexual pain are dyspareunia and vulvodynia. *Dyspareunia* is defined as recurrent or persistent pain with sexual activity that causes significant distress or interpersonal conflict. Up to 19% of women in the United States suffer from dyspareunia (West et al. 2004). Globally, the World Health Organization reports rates of 8–22% (Mitchell et al. 2017; Steege and Zolnoun 2009). Painful intercourse is sometimes further characterized as *vulvodynia*—chronic genital pain of unknown aetiology most often described as burning pain, lasting more than three months, that may or may not be associated with sexual intercourse (Sorensen et al. 2018; Goldstein et al. 2016).

There are several classifications of dyspareunia: *entry dyspareunia*—pain with initial or attempted penetration of the introitus; *deep dyspareunia*—pain with deeper vaginal penetration; *primary dyspareunia*—occurring with first sexual debut and thereafter; *secondary dyspareunia*—beginning some time after previously painless sexual activity (Sorensen et al. 2018; Seehusen et al. 2014). Secondary dyspareunia is often associated with specific triggering events such as trauma or exposure to infection (Sorensen et al. 2018).

S. Kellogg Spadt · L. Tannenbaum (✉)
Center for Pelvic Medicine, Bryn Mawr, PA, USA
e-mail: ldt38@drexel.edu

© Springer Nature Switzerland AG 2021   97
A. Rantell (ed.), *Sexual Function and Pelvic Floor Dysfunction*,
https://doi.org/10.1007/978-3-030-63843-6_9

Table 9.1 Demonstrates the differentiating factors between dyspareunia and vulvodynia

Dyspareunia	Vulvodynia
• Can be acute or chronic • Associated with intercourse • Occurs at the entrance to the vagina, deeper in the vaginal canal and in the pelvis	• Chronic • May or may not be associated with intercourse • Can occur spontaneously without provocation • Limited to the vulva and vaginal entrance, or introitus

Although dyspareunia can be a symptom of vulvodynia, differentiating factors have been summarized in Table 9.1 (Sorensen et al. 2018). Factors associated with the development of dyspareunia include vaginal dryness and inadequate lubrication secondary to arousal disorders or vulvovaginal atrophy, and childbirth—perineal stretching, lacerations, operative vaginal delivery, and episiotomy can all result in sclerotic healing and subsequent entry or deep dyspareunia (Sorensen et al. 2018; Seehusen et al. 2014).

Vulvodynia can be *localized*—limited to the vulvar vestibule around the hymenal ring at the entrance of the vagina; *generalized*—affecting the entire vulvar area and can be associated with pain that is intermittent, persistent, constant, immediate, or delayed. Associated factors in the development of vulvodynia include other pain syndromes such as fibromyalgia or irritable bowel syndrome, genetic and hormonal influences, inflammation, musculoskeletal or neurologic mechanisms, psychosocial factors, and structural defects (Sorensen et al. 2018).

Both dyspareunia and vulvodynia can result from several conditions including vulvovaginal skin conditions and dermatoses, such as lichen sclerosus or lichen planus, genitourinary infections, sexually transmitted infections, endometriosis, and pelvic floor dysfunction (PFD) (Sorensen et al. 2018; Mitchell et al. 2017). Deep dyspareunia is often associated with visceral disorders such as interstitial cystitis, pelvic inflammatory disease, endometriosis, adhesions, pelvic congestion syndrome, and fibroids (Sorensen et al. 2018). Dyspareunia can also lead to other sexual disorders such as decreased libido, decreased arousal, and anorgasmia causing strain within the sexual relationship (Mitchell et al. 2017; Seehusen et al. 2014).

9.2 Desire, Arousal, and Orgasm Disorders

Female Sexual Dysfunction (FSD) is common and affects approximately 44% of women at least once in their life, with the highest prevalence in midlife; 12% of women report it as distressing (Kusturiss and Kellogg Spadt 2017; Paykel 2018). The World Health Organization defines sexual dysfunction as "the various ways in which an individual is unable to participate in a sexual relationship the way they would wish" (Beckmann and Ling 2019). Unfortunately FSD remains underdiagnosed and undertreated by health care providers (Kusturiss and Kellogg Spadt 2017).

FSD includes dyspareunia and *vaginismus*—an involuntary contraction of the pelvic floor muscles prohibiting entry into the vagina, in addition to non-painful conditions—hypoactive sexual desire disorder (HSDD), female arousal disorder (FAD), and female orgasmic disorder (FOD) (Beckmann and Ling 2019; Kusturiss and Kellogg Spadt 2017; Paykel 2018). The PRESIDE (Prevalence of Female Sexual Problems Associated with Distress and Determinants of Treatment Seeking) study published in 2008 reported that decreased sexual desire was the most prevalent distressing sexual dysfunction, affecting approximately 38.7% of women, followed by low arousal at 26.1%, and difficulty with orgasm at 20.5% (Kusturiss and Kellogg Spadt 2017; Paykel 2018). Diagnosis of any FSD requires the presence of three criteria: symptoms must be persistent or recurrent, it must cause personal on interpersonal distress, and the symptoms cannot be caused by another disorder, medical condition, medication, or substance abuse (Paykel 2018).

Female desire and arousal disorder is additionally based on having at least three diagnostic criteria of a possible six: (1) decreased sexual activity due to absent or diminished interest, (2) lack of erotic or sexual thoughts and fantasies, (3) little or no interest in initiating sexual activity or responding to same from partner, (4) sexual excitement or pleasure is reduced in most (75–100%) sexual encounters, (5) internal or external sexual cues fail to spark interest or arousal, and (6) genital or nongenital sensations are greatly reduced in 75–100% of sexual encounters (Kusturiss and Kellogg Spadt 2017; Paykel 2018).

Female orgasmic disorder (FOD) is defined as marked delay, infrequency, or absence of orgasm following a normal excitement phase, or greatly reduced intensity of sensations caused by orgasm. For diagnosis, symptoms must be present for a minimum of 6 months, during approximately 75–100% of sexual encounters, and significant distress must be present (Kusturiss and Kellogg Spadt 2017). Prevalence ranges from 4% to 42% based on various studies (Kusturiss and Kellogg Spadt 2017). Women with FOD often have sexual interest and/or arousal disorder as well (Beckmann and Ling 2019; Paykel 2018).

Treatment of FSD is based on aetiology and may include sex therapy with a certified therapist, use of pharmacologic intervention or hormone therapy, and/or use of sexual devices (Beckmann and Ling 2019).

9.3 Pelvic Floor Dysfunction

The pelvic floor muscles, known collectively as the levator ani muscles, consist of the superficial (transverse perineal, bulbospongiosus, and ischiocavernosus) muscles and the deep (pubococcygeus, iliococcygeus, obturator internus, and coccygeus) muscles. Their function is to provide direct support to the viscera of the urinary, genital, and rectal compartments of the pelvis and to provide secondary postural stabilization to the bony pelvis. Normal function of the pelvic floor musculature is essential in maintaining appropriate support and function of the pelvic organs and contributes to adequate urination, defecation, and sexual response (Prendergast and Rummer 2016; JM1 et al. 2014).

Pelvic floor dysfunction (PFD) refers to conditions in which the pelvic floor muscular support system is functioning abnormally (Butrick 2009). The term low-tone pelvic floor dysfunction denotes weak, underactive, and hypotonic muscles that cannot attain or maintain adequate contraction, leading to symptoms of incontinence, altered sexual sensation, and pelvic organ prolapse (Faubion et al. 2012; Meister et al. 2019). Common complaints include pressure, heaviness, and aching that can be exacerbated by exertion, elimination, prolonged sitting, and coitus (Weiss et al. 2012).

Another type of pelvic floor muscle dysfunction results from weak pelvic floor muscles that cannot attain or maintain adequate relaxation, and become overactive, hypertonic, spastic, and shortened. The term high-tone pelvic floor dysfunction describes this phenomenon and is also referred to as tension myalgia of the pelvic floor and vaginismus. This type of dysfunction is prevalent, is commonly associated with prohibitive sexual pain in women (Faubion et al. 2012; Kellogg Spadt and Kusturiss 2019; Moldwin and Fariello 2013) and is discussed further in Chap. 13.

High-tone pelvic floor dysfunction can result from several etiologies, including: muscle or nerve trauma during childbirth; urinary, vaginal, or uterine infections; adhesions and surgical trauma; instability in the sacroiliac joint, hip, or spine; accidental fall or injury; postural stressors such as prolonged standing or sitting, and asymmetric skeletal overload in certain vocations, intense or elite athleticism, short leg syndrome or gait disturbances; and history of sexual abuse. High-tone pelvic floor dysfunction can present with symptoms of: penetrative dyspareunia, frequency, urgency, dysuria, urinary retention, faecal retention and/or constipation (Weiss et al. 2012; Seehusen et al. 2014; Prendergast and Rummer 2016; Faubion et al. 2012; Moldwin and Fariello 2013).

A characteristic of high-tone pelvic floor dysfunction is the occurrence of hyper-irritable areas within the muscles called myofascial trigger points (Moldwin and Fariello 2013). Active myofascial trigger points are associated with either local or referred pain patterns and can often reproduce the patient's complaint of pain. For instance, a trigger point within the pubococcygeus muscle can create a tender area with direct palpation of the muscle or it could refer pain to the introitus, creating sensations of burning that could be mistaken for a vaginal infection (Goldstein and Kellogg-Spadt 2018). If left untreated, myofascial trigger points and progressive muscle hypertonicity can result in compression of deeper neural structures (e.g. pudendal nerve) and cause neuropathic symptoms (Prendergast and Rummer 2016; Kellogg Spadt and Kusturiss 2019; Moldwin and Fariello 2013). Prevalence estimates of pelvic floor muscle-related pain disorders vary widely from 14% to 78% (Meister et al. 2019).

High-tone pelvic floor dysfunction can occur as a result of an injury or accident affecting the hip or back—types of injuries for which athletic or infirm women may be particularly vulnerable. With injury to the upper pelvic stabilizers, there is increased metabolic activity within the pelvic floor muscles causing the muscle to spasm. Over time, the muscles become fibrotic, with decreased flexibility and impaired relaxation. The increased muscle tension triggers pain and more reflex tightening, and the vicious cycle of pelvic floor hypertonus begins (Kellogg Spadt and Kusturiss 2019; Hartmann and Sarton 2014).

A lesser-known antecedent of PFD is chronic irritation of the viscera as is seen in bladder, bowel, and genital disorders (Prendergast and Rummer 2016; Moldwin and Fariello 2013). For example, a woman who has hypersensitivity associated with urogenital conditions such as chronic cystitis, chronic yeast infections, endometriosis, urethritis, provoked vestibulodynia, or interstitial cystitis may be at risk for comorbid high-tone pelvic floor dysfunction (Weiss et al. 2012). The vagina, vestibule, urethra, and bladder all originate from the same embryologic tissue, and share many nerve, muscle and receptor similarities, explaining the coexistence and correlation with these conditions (Steege and Zolnoun 2009).

Due to the multifactorial aetiology of dyspareunia, pelvic pain, and PFD, it is critically important for clinicians to perform a comprehensive and methodical evaluation of the woman who presents with these issues (West et al. 2004). It should consist of a medical history and a physical, psychological, and pelvic floor muscle assessment, the latter being too often neglected during the evaluation of pelvic disorders by non-specialists, as few clinicians are trained to examine these muscles in their basic education programmes (Weiss et al. 2012).

9.4 History Taking

Obtaining history and completing a thorough examination allows the time to gather information and establish a trusting rapport. Therapeutic effects of the provider–patient relationship should not be overlooked and the overall goal should be to validate the patient's symptoms, understand pertinent history, and to educate and reassure the patient (Sorensen et al. 2018; Goldstein et al. 2016). The provider should maintain direct eye contact and sit if possible to convey to the patient that her issue is important and worthy of time and attention (Kusturiss and Kellogg Spadt 2017).

Detailed history includes pain characteristics if applicable (location, duration, exacerbating factors, triggers), associated symptoms such as bowel, bladder, or musculoskeletal symptoms; sexual behaviour; psychological history; comorbid medical problems; current health status; medications; previous treatments; and history of physical or sexual abuse (Sorensen et al. 2018; Kusturiss and Kellogg Spadt 2017). It may be helpful to establish general medical-surgical and musculoskeletal history first before progressing to the more sensitive gynecologic, obstetric, and comprehensive sexual history (Sorensen et al. 2018; Seehusen et al. 2014; Goldstein et al. 2016).

9.4.1 Medical History

A patient's narrative of her illness provides essential information to determine the correct diagnosis of the presenting complaint. However, a woman's experience of pelvic dysfunction and/or sexual pain is often more complicated and may be less straightforward than other medical conditions. In addition, an affected woman may experience embarrassment, shame, guilt, loss of self-esteem, frustration, depression, and anxiety surrounding sexuality. Therefore, it is highly important for a clinician to use communication skills that enhance openness, comfort, trust, and confidence (see Table 9.2) (Goldstein and Kellogg-Spadt 2018; Sorensen et al. 2018).

In general, a woman with sexual pain will see several clinicians in her search to find appropriate care for her condition (Bornstein et al. 2015). She may feel patronized, marginalized, and angry from previous encounters. It is important for the clinician to address these feelings in order to establish a constructive and trusting relationship. Privacy and assurances of confidentiality are essential when conducting the interview. Some patients may want a spouse, sexual partner, relative, or friend present during the interview or examination. While this may allow the patient to feel more comfortable, it might also inhibit the patient from disclosing pertinent aspects of her medical, social, relationship, or sexual history. When possible, there should be some time allotted for the patient and the clinician to discuss a sexual history privately (Goldstein et al. 2016; Kellogg Spadt and Kusturiss 2019).

It is important to ask direct questions to obtain specific information, such as medication usage, and equally essential to ask open-ended questions that allow a patient to describe her experience of the condition without being interrupted (Bornstein et al. 2015). A useful prompt for this narrative might be, "Complete this sentence… I was feeling fine until…". Throughout the whole process, displaying empathy, understanding, and acceptance is vital. Repeating the information back to the patient to confirm the accuracy of her history is also an important component (Goldstein and Kellogg-Spadt 2018; Goldstein et al. 2016). If there are several different complaints, determine which she feels is her chief complaint. If there is not enough time to focus on a specific complaint during a single visit, the patient should be reassured of the importance of her problem and scheduled for a follow-up appointment to address that issue alone (Goldstein and Kellogg-Spadt 2018; Kellogg Spadt and Kusturiss 2019).

In cases of sexual pain, validated questionnaires can be used for screening and to aid diagnosis. The female sexual function index, female sexual distress scale, the

Table 9.2 Suggested skills for an optimal professional relationship with a patient/client

Ensuring the patient of confidentiality/privacy
Finding a balance between being formal/informal during patient interviewing and ask both closed- and open-ended questions
Provide ample time for a new patient to remain clothed during the first part of the interview, as she narrates (uninterrupted) her experience of the condition
If the patient becomes emotional, allow for moments of silence, as can be cathartic for her; allowing her the space to express her feelings and feeling valued in the clinician–patient relationship
Asking while displaying empathy, understanding, and acceptance
Considering patient requests for a support person to attend the meeting(s) (although some history may not be revealed with another person present)
Repeating some of the information back to the patient in order to confirm the accuracy of your understanding to her
Reacting in an appropriate manner (i.e. in a calm, accepting, and professional manner) to the content of the discussion

McGill pain questionnaire, or the Patient Reported Outcomes Measurement Information System (PROMIS) can be efficient tools for clinicians with limited time to collect information on the quality and intensity of the patient's pain and the impact it has on their lives (Sorensen et al. 2018; Kusturiss and Kellogg Spadt 2017; Paykel 2018). A recently developed validated instrument, the vulvar pain assessment questionnaire can also be extremely useful in the evaluation of dyspareunia as well as following progress of treatment (Goldstein et al. 2016; Dargie et al. 2016).

After both an accurate history of present illness and chief complaint have been established, additional information (see Table 9.3) should be gathered that may help the clinician narrow the differential diagnosis (Goldstein and Kellogg-Spadt 2018; Goldstein et al. 2016).

9.4.2 Medication History

More than 90% of women take prescription medications (Goldstein et al. 2016), therefore, a discussion of the most commonly prescribed medications is warranted. It is important to note that patients frequently do not disclose use of herbal

Table 9.3 Specific questions to ask while obtaining history

– Pain characteristics if present, such as time since onset, duration, location, quality, elicitors, intensity
– Musculoskeletal history, persistent joint pain, orthopaedic diagnosis or surgery. Injury/falls affecting the lumbo-pelvic-hip region and/or to the tailbone and sacrum. Any history of scoliosis
– Description of childhood and adult athleticism, current athletic workout programme, competitions, details of injuries
– Medical history—chronic health conditions such as diabetes, hypertension, and hypothyroid
– Details regarding previous labours—types of delivery, lacerations, complications; GYN surgeries; hormone status—reproductive age, peri- or post-menopausal
– Bowel and bladder function: frequency, urgency, constipation, etc., history of UTI/rUTI, impact on daily activities
– Sexuality: desire, arousal, orgasm, frequency of and satisfaction/distress with sexual activity
– Current relationship: strengths, degree of effect on their relationship, how they cope as a couple, emotional and non-sexual physical intimacy
– Thoughts, emotions, behaviours, and couple interactions that accompany the pain experience (i.e. negative partner responses)
– Comorbid mental health conditions and treatments; anxiety, depression, substance abuse
– Previous treatment attempts and outcomes
– Medications—antibiotics, contraceptives, antidepressants, anxiolytics, hormone therapy, anticonvulsants
– Home and work status
– Trauma including abuse and neglect, and any nonconsensual/negative sexual experiences
– Standardized self-report questionnaires (e.g. female sexual function index) may be useful for making comparisons with clinical norms or to track treatment progress

supplements to clinicians; thus, it is important to ask about herbs, vitamins, and complementary or alternative therapies when inquiring about medication history (Goldstein and Kellogg-Spadt 2018).

Antibiotics are one of the most common prescription medications used by women. While antibiotics do not directly cause sexual pain, long-term exposure does predispose women to alteration in the gut and vaginal flora, and chronic yeast infections, which may be a causative agent of the pain. Combined hormonal contraceptives (CHCs) (e.g. oral contraceptives, transdermal patch, vaginal ring) are the second most common prescription medication used by reproductive-aged women. The use of these agents is highly associated with *vestibulodynia*, the most common cause of dyspareunia in premenopausal women, characterized by severe pain upon touch of the vestibule or attempt at vaginal entry, along with vestibular erythema. Although not all women who use combined hormonal contraceptives develop sexual pain, in at least one case-control study, women who used oral contraceptives were 9.3 times more likely to develop vestibulodynia than controls (Brewer et al. 2007). Several authors suggest that women who use or have used low-dose ethinyl estradiol oral contraceptives are more likely to develop vestibulodynia. The proposed mechanism linking CHCs to sexual pain suggests that CHC use results in elevated sex hormone binding globulin (SHBG) and decreased free circulating testosterone, which may result in dysfunction of the androgen-dependent mucin glands and atrophy of the endodermal mucosa of the vulvar vestibule, placing a woman at risk for chronic inflammation and dyspareunia (Goldstein et al. 2016; Dargie et al. 2016).

In addition, approximately 20% of reproductive-aged women use prescription medications for anxiety and depression. The most common cause of reduced libido is depression; concomitantly, psychotropic medications are frequently implicated as a cause of alterations in female sexual desire and lubrication. Both of these can contribute to dyspareunia due to their adverse effects on vaginal lubrication and sexual arousal (Beckmann and Ling 2019; Goldstein et al. 2016; Glover et al. 2004).

Lastly, many medications can be used to treat sexual health issues and pelvic floor dysfunction. Questions regarding previous use and efficacy of medications such as muscle relaxants, suppositories, injections, Botox, etc., as well as herbal supplements should be reviewed (Goldstein and Kellogg-Spadt 2018; Kellogg Spadt and Kusturiss 2019).

9.5   Physical Exam

All women with pelvic and/or sexual complaints should undergo a thorough physical examination of the pelvic floor muscles in addition to routine gynaecological evaluation. While this exam focuses primarily on the urogenital system, additional organ systems may need to be assessed depending on information obtained during the medical history (Goldstein et al. 2016). For those health care professionals that are not confident performing full internal examinations, a basic assessment on perineal health and skin integrity in the vulval region should be performed prior to review by an appropriately trained clinician.

It is important to recognize that some aspects of a patient's medical history may need validation. For instance, it is common for a woman with pain related to pelvic floor muscle dysfunction to self-report a history of "chronic yeast infections". In reality, this may or may not be the cause of her symptoms if the diagnosis has not been validated by clinical microscopy or laboratory culture (Bouchard et al. 2002). In addition, some women have a difficult time localizing sources of pelvic pain. They may incorrectly identify the location of their pain localizing it to the urethra or vagina while an examination reveals that the pain is originating from the pelvic floor muscles (Goldstein and Kellogg-Spadt 2018).

The goal of the physical exam is to gather data to determine the aetiology of the chief complaint. It is essential to discuss and explain the process in detail before, during, and after the evaluation is performed so the patient is involved and has clear expectations through each step of the assessment (Sorensen et al. 2018). It can be beneficial for the patient to watch the physical exam with a mirror to establish common nomenclature for the parts of the urogenital system and to show findings that are related to her experience. This type of educational exam can also assist her in monitoring her own treatment progress, in addition to increasing her comfort and perception of control (Weiss et al. 2012; Seehusen et al. 2014). In cases of sexual pain, if the examiner can identify the correct location and reproduce a woman's pain, she feels validated as this shows her that her sexual pain is real and has a physical origin. It also inspires confidence that the practitioner will be able to treat her pain (Goldstein and Kellogg-Spadt 2018; Goldstein et al. 2016; Kellogg Spadt and Kusturiss 2019).

9.5.1 Vulvoscopy

During colposcopic examination of the vulva, commonly referred to vulvoscopy, important findings that can be observed include: infection, trauma, atrophy, and dermatitis (Sorensen et al. 2018; Goldstein et al. 2016). If unavailable, an external visual assessment can be performed with or without the use of magnification. Specifically, the observer should note any inflammation, induration, excoriation, fissures, ulceration, lichenification, hypopigmentation, hyperpigmentation, scarring, or architectural changes, which may be evidence for dermatologic disease of the vulva. While erythema is a nonspecific finding, intense redness near the ostia of the Bartholin and Skene glands is suggestive of vestibulodynia (Goldstein et al. 2016).

9.5.2 Sensory Exam

A key component of a pelvic pain evaluation is the genital sensory exam. This is performed using a moistened cotton swab (called the "Q-tip test") to determine if there are areas that exhibit an abnormal pain response. This exam should be performed systematically to ensure that all areas of the anogenital region are tested

(Sorensen et al. 2018; Goldstein et al. 2016). Undue discomfort should be avoided to minimize guarding, which could limit a thorough examination.

Initially, the medial thigh, buttocks, and mons pubis are palpated. These areas are typically not painful and this allows the patient to get comfortable with this exam. Then the labia majora, clitoral prepuce, perineum, and interlabial sulci should be evaluated. Pain in these areas would suggest a process that is affecting the whole anogenital region including vulvar dermatoses, vulvovaginal infections, or neuropathic processes such as pudendal neuralgia. The labia minora are then gently palpated, followed by the medial labia minora lateral to Hart's line, which is the boundary of the vulvar vestibule (Goldstein et al. 2016; Kusturiss and Kellogg Spadt 2017).

The cotton swab is then used to gently palpate the vestibule at five locations: at the ostia of the Skene glands (lateral to the urethra), at the ostia of the Bartholin glands (5 and 7 o'clock on the vestibule), and at 6 o'clock at the posterior fourchette. The patient is asked to grade the pain on a scale of 0–10. If the pain elicited with the Q-tip touch is localized to the vestibule, it is important to determine if the pain affects the entire vaginal opening or just the posterior portion of vestibule because pain throughout the entire vestibule may be associated with pathology within the tissue of the vestibule, whereas pain confined to the posterior vestibule (the "5, 6, 7 o'clock positions") suggests that the pain might be associated with hypertonic (overactive) pelvic floor muscle dysfunction (Goldstein and Kellogg-Spadt 2018; Goldstein et al. 2016; King et al. 2014). This is demonstrated in Fig. 9.1 below taken from Sorensen et al. (2018).

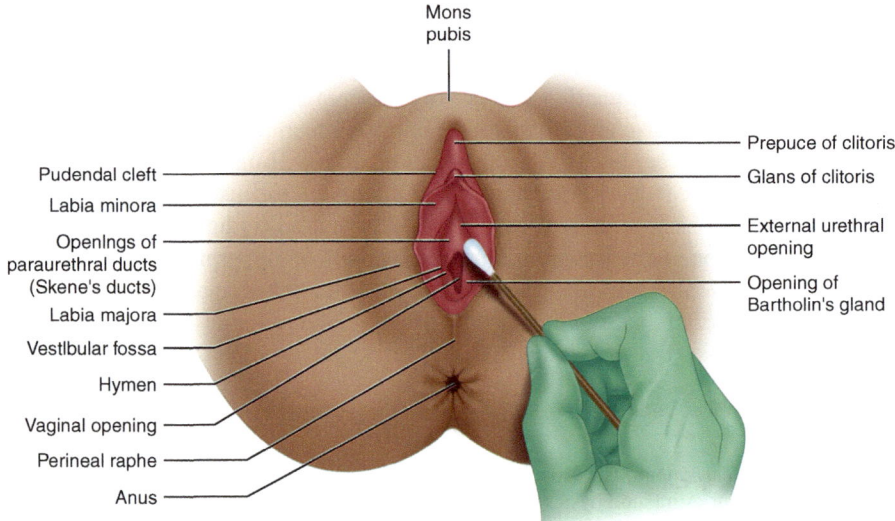

Fig. 9.1 Demonstration of Q-tip sensory testing. Source: Sorensen J, Bautista K E, Lamvu G, et al. (March 27, 2018) Evaluation and Treatment of Female Sexual Pain: A Clinical Review. Cureus 10(3): e2379. doi:10.7759/cureus.2379

9.5.3 Manual Exam

A manual exam is then performed. The examiner's single index finger is inserted through the hymenal ring without touching the vestibule. The urethra and bladder trigone are gently palpated. Intrinsic tenderness of the urethra may be suggestive of a urethral diverticulum while tenderness of the bladder may be suggestive of inter-stitial cystitis. The pelvic floor muscles are then palpated for hypertonicity. Sensations of pain with palpation (as opposed to the normal sensation of pressure), weakness with attempted contraction, inability to relax the muscles, or identifica-tion of tender points in the muscles can be evidence of PFD (Goldstein and Kellogg-Spadt 2018; Goldstein et al. 2016; Prendergast and Rummer 2016; Kellogg Spadt and Kusturiss 2019).

The ischial spine is then located and the pudendal nerve is palpated as it enters Alcock's canal. Tenderness of the pudendal nerve is suggestive of pudendal neural-gia or pudendal nerve entrapment. Next, if the patient tolerated the muscular exam, a bimanual examination is performed to assess the uterus and adnexa (ovaries and fallopian tubes). Abnormalities in the size, shape, or contour may be indicative of a leiomyoma (fibroid). A diffusely enlarged, "boggy" and tender uterus may be evi-dence of adenomyosis. Tenderness of the adnexa can often be a sign of a sexually transmitted infection, pelvic inflammatory disease, or endometriosis. A rectovaginal examination is then performed to assess the rectovaginal septum and the posterior cul-de-sac. Thickening or nodularity of the septum, nodularity of the uterosacral ligaments, or obliteration of the posterior cul-de-sac can be suggestive of endome-triosis. Traumatic neuromas can also be a source of significant pain in women who have had prior vaginal surgery, including repair of lacerations or episiotomies incurred during childbirth (Goldstein et al. 2016).

Pelvic floor muscle coordination can be assessed by asking the woman to con-tract her muscles around the examiner's gloved fingers, hold for a count of five, and then relax the muscles and produce a "bulge" movement. If the woman is unable to contract, relax, or bulge and demonstrates any pain in the pelvic floor muscles, she should be triaged by the health care provider for a detailed assessment and pelvic floor muscle treatment plan. This is accomplished by a referral to an experienced manual physical therapist with specialized pelvic floor training (Goldstein and Kellogg-Spadt 2018; Kellogg Spadt and Kusturiss 2019). Lastly, the woman's pos-ture, alignment, gait patterns, movement or the sacroiliac joint, spine, and hip should also be evaluated, noting limitations in range of motion, and strength and joint integrity (Goldstein and Kellogg-Spadt 2018; Kellogg Spadt and Kusturiss 2019).

It should be noted that many women are treated for sexual pain suboptimally by well-meaning clinicians. They are given medication for yeast infections, hormonal creams for dry irritated tissue, oral pain medications, and counselling for anxiety. Pelvic floor muscle assessment and subsequent referral for physical therapy is often the "missing piece" of a comprehensive plan of care for sexual pain, and is critical for facilitating long-lasting sexual health (Weiss et al. 2012).

9.5.4 Speculum Exam

A speculum exam of the vagina is the next step in the physical examination. In general, a paediatric-sized Graves speculum should be used and all efforts should be used to insert the speculum through the hymeneal ring without touching the vulvar vestibule. Initially, the vagina should be examined for evidence of abnormal vaginal discharge. A cotton swab should be used to collect some discharge for pH testing, wet mount, and potassium hydroxide (KOH) prep. In addition, a culture should be obtained and sent for microscopy, culture, and sensitivity. Important findings while visualizing the vagina include atrophy, erythema, erosions, ulcerations, abnormal discharge, or synechiae (Goldstein et al. 2016).

In cases of pelvic organ prolapse, a single blade of the speculum can be used to inspect the vaginal walls systematically—anterior, apical, and posterior assessment—identifying defects in each compartment. Asking the patient to "bear down", or Valsalva, can induce the maximum prolapse to allow for classification: stage 0, normal position, no prolapse; stage 1, descent is >1 cm above the hymen; stage 2, descent to hymen is ≤1 cm; stage 3, descent is past hymen but protrudes less than or equal to the total vaginal length; and stage 4, complete eversion. Most prolapses are asymptomatic; however, advanced prolapse may cause incomplete emptying of the bladder or rectum requiring patients to splint the vagina in order to void or defecate. A rectovaginal exam may be required to assess for enterocele, posterior wall defect, and pelvic muscle and anal sphincter strength (Beckmann and Ling 2019).

9.6 Summary

Women's health care providers have a paramount role in assessing sexual function, urogenital conditions, and pelvic floor disorders. A comprehensive psychosocial evaluation must be included in order to fully understand the experience of women who suffer from these issues. This should be followed by a detailed history and systematic gynecologic, urologic, and pelvic floor examination. When pelvic floor dysfunction is identified, the patient should be triaged for specialized pelvic floor physical therapy. Based on findings, referrals to mental health practitioners, relationship counsellors, sex therapists, or support groups may be appropriate. With adequate knowledge and thorough assessment, health care providers can identify pelvic floor and sexual disorders and use multimodal approaches and interdisciplinary referrals to optimally address the health concerns of women (Goldstein and Kellogg-Spadt 2018; Sorensen et al. 2018).

References

Beckmann CR, Ling FW (2019) Human sexuality. In: Obstetrics & gynecology, 8th edn. Wolters Kluwer, Philadelphia, PA

Bornstein J, Goldstein AT, Stockdale CK et al (2015) ISSVD, ISSWSH, and IPPS consensus terminology and classification of persistent vulvar pain and vulvodynia. J Sex Med 13:607–612

Bouchard C, Brisson J, Fortier M et al (2002) Use of oral contraceptive pills and vulvar vestibulitis: a case-control study. Am J Epidemiol 156:254–261

Brewer ME, White WM, Klein FA et al (2007) Validity of pelvic pain, urgency, and frequency questionnaire in patients with interstitial cystitis/painful bladder syndrome. Urology 70:646–649

Butrick CW (2009) Pathophysiology of the pelvic floor hypertonic disorders. Obstet Gynecol Clin N Am 36(3):699–705

Dargie E, Holden RR, Pukall CF (2016) The vulvar pain assessment questionnaire inventory. Pain 157(12):2672–2686

Faubion SS, Shudter LT, Bharucha AE (2012) Recognition and management of nonrelaxing pelvic floor dysfunction. Mayo Clin Proc 87(2):187–193

Glover DD, Rybeck BF, Tracy TS (2004) Medication use in rural gynecologic population: prescription, over-the-counter, and herbal medicines. Am J Obstet Gynecol 190:351–357

Goldstein AT, Kellogg-Spadt S (2018) Medical management of dyspareunia and vulvovaginal pain. In: Goldstein I, Clayton A, Goldstein A, Kim N, Kingsberg S (eds) Textbook of female function and dysfunction. Wiley and Sons, New York, NY

Goldstein AT, Pukall CF, Brown C, Bergeron S, Stein A, Kellogg-Spadt S (2016) Vulvodynia: assessment and treatment. J Sex Med 13(4):572–590

Hartmann D, Sarton J (2014) Chronic pelvic floor dysfunction. Best Pract Res Clin Obstet Gynaecol 28(7):977–990

Kellogg Spadt S, Kusturiss E (2019) Pelvic floor function. In: Menopause practice: a clinician's guide, 6th edn. NAMS, Pepper Pike, OH, pp 90–93

King M, Rubin R, Goldstein A (2014) Current uses of surgery for the treatment of genital pain. Curr Sex Health Rep 6(4):252–258. https://doi.org/10.1007/s11930-014-0032-8

Kusturiss E, Kellogg Spadt S (2017) Women's sexual health. In: Alexander IM, Johnson-Mallard V, Kostas-Polston EA, Ingram Fogel C, Fugate Woods N (eds) Women's health care in advanced practice nursing, 2nd edn. Springer Publishing Company, New York, NY

Meister MR, Sutcliffe S, Ghetti C et al (2019) Development of a standardized, reproducible screening examination for assessment of pelvic floor myofascial pain. Am J Obstet Gynecol 220:255.e1–255.e9

Mitchell KR, Geary R, Graham CA et al (2017) Painful sex (dyspareunia) in women: prevalence and associated factors in a British population probability survey. BJOG 124(11):1689–1697

Moldwin RM, Fariello JY (2013) Myofascial trigger points of the pelvic floor: associations with urological pain syndromes and treatment strategies including injection therapy. Curr Urol Rep 14(5):409–417

Paykel JM (2018) Integrative treatment of female sexual dysfunction. In: Bartlik B, Espinosa G, Mindes J (eds) Integrative sexual health. Oxford University Press, New York, NY

Prendergast SA, Rummer EH (2016) Pelvic pain explained. Rowan and Littlefied, New York, NY

Seehusen DA, Baird DC, Boda DV (2014) Dyspareunia in women. Am Fam Physician 90(7):465–470

Sorensen J, Bautista KE, Lamvu G, Feranec J (2018) Evaluation and treatment of female sexual pain: a clinical review. Cureus 10(3):e2379

Steege JF, Zolnoun DA (2009) Evaluation and treatment of dyspareunia. Obstet Gynecol 113(5):1124–1136

Weiss PM, Rich J, Swisher E (2012) Pelvic floor spasm: the missing link in chronic pelvic pain. Contemp Ob/Gyn 57:38–46

West SL, Vinikoor LC, Zolnoun D (2004) A systematic review of the literature on female sexual dysfunction prevalence and predictors. Annu Rev Sex Res 15:40–172

Wu JM, Vaughan CP, Goode PS, Redden DT, Burgio KL, Richter HE, Markland AD (2014 Jan) Prevalence and trends of symptomatic pelvic floor disorders in U.S. women. Obstet Gynecol 123(1):141–148

Subjective and Objective Measure of Sexual Function in PFD

10

Sushma Srikrishna and Angie Rantell

10.1 Introduction

Sexual health is a state of physical, emotional, mental, and social well-being in relation to sexuality; it is not merely the absence of disease, dysfunction, or infirmity (WHO 2006). Pelvic floor disorders (PFD), including urinary (UI), and pelvic organ prolapse (POP) often adversely affect sexual health (Rogers et al. 2001; Pauls et al. 2006). Up to 60% of sexually active women attending urogynaecology clinics report sexual dysfunction (SD) (Pauls et al. 2006; Temml et al. 2000). Sexual problems commonly described in women with POP or SUI include disorders of desire, arousal, orgasm, and dyspareunia.

Sexual satisfaction depends not just on the physical act of coitus but on a more complex interplay of other aspects such as emotional well-being, interaction with a partner, self-image, and self-confidence, all of which can be impaired by pelvic floor dysfunction (PFD). This chapter aims to review the objective and subjective outcome measures that may be used in the clinical assessment of SD in women with PFD.

10.2 Clinical History and Examination

As demonstrated in Chap. 9, assessment of sexual function should start with a complete history followed by thorough examination. Initial assessment should focus on symptoms experienced by women, followed by a detailed medical history with a particular focus on identifying other risk factors, e.g. chronic constipation, collagen disorders (benign joint hypermobility/Ehlers–Danlos syndrome), and familial history of prolapse. A vaginal examination should be performed to assess for prolapse.

S. Srikrishna · A. Rantell (✉)
Urogynaecology Department, King's College Hospital, London, UK
e-mail: sushmasrikrishna@nhs.net; angela.rantell@nhs.net

© Springer Nature Switzerland AG 2021
A. Rantell (ed.), *Sexual Function and Pelvic Floor Dysfunction*,
https://doi.org/10.1007/978-3-030-63843-6_10

There are many different staging and grading systems in the literature but the Pelvic Organ Prolapse Quantification System (POP-Q) is the recommended method. The choice of the woman's position during examination, e.g. left lateral (Sims), supine, standing or lithotomy is that which can best demonstrate POP in that patient and which the woman can confirm as the maximal extent she has perceived e.g. by use of a mirror or digital palpation.

If there are urinary symptoms, it may be necessary to consider urinalysis ± a midstream specimen of urine (MSU), post-void residual urine volume testing, urodynamic investigations, or a renal ultrasound scan. If there are bowel symptoms, consider ano-rectal manometry, defaecating proctography, and an endo-anal ultrasound scan. A trans-vaginal ultrasound scan will also help to rule out any pelvic mass that may add to or cause symptoms on prolapse, particularly in women for whom bimanual examination is suboptimal due to body habitus.

10.3   Assessment of Quality of Life

Patient reported outcome measures (PROMs) are specifically validated questionnaires that can be used to identify or diagnose a particular dysfunction, assess the severity or impact on HRQL and measure improvement or satisfaction with treatment (Althof and Symonds 2007; Rogers et al. 2013). They are usually self-administered and can be completed by a patient in her own time prior to assessment, encouraging reflection on symptoms and aiding discussion; however, due to the sensitive nature of SF some women may not wish to complete them. Questionnaires measure 'subjective' information in an 'objective' fashion and as such they provide a reproducible method for evaluating female sexual function. The use of validated questionnaires assures data that are reliable, quantifiable, and reproducible.

The development of quality of life questionnaires is a complex and lengthy process. It generally involves an initial stage of item generation, which is based on reviews of the literature and subject/expert opinions gained from focus groups/interviews. This is followed by item reduction where subjects and experts express preferences to topics and questions and these views are then translated during an expert meeting to generate a questionnaire. This is then piloted in a small group of subjects prior to more formal testing to confirm content, face, criterion and construct validity and reliability of the measure.

Given this arduous process, there are very few truly high quality questionnaires assessing SF in women. The International Consultation on Incontinence (ICI) have performed repeated literature searches over the years as part of the assessment chapter of the textbook to identify questionnaires to assess PROMS. These tools are then subject to a stringent review of the reliability and validity of the measure and the quality of the evidence supporting its development and use in clinical populations. Based on the levels of evidence, the ICI then make recommendations on which tools to use. Gradings are from A+ to C and those with an A+ rating are highly recommended (Abrams et al. 2017).

Quality of Life (QoL) questionnaires and symptom-specific questionnaires can be useful in the clinical setting, particularly when women report a variety of bladder, bowel, and sexual dysfunction symptoms. There are many validated questionnaires available to assess QoL in women with PFD, e.g. The King's Health Questionnaire (KHQ) and Pelvic organ prolapse symptom questionnaire (POP-S). The ICI have developed modular questionnaires that are available and free to download to all clinicians at http://iciq.net/.

Validated questionnaires utilized to assess sexual function in women with PFD may be generalized or condition-specific. Generalized questionnaires focusing on sexual function were designed to evaluate sexual function in a general population and not specifically in women with PFD. These types of questionnaires may not be sensitive enough to detect differences due to the disease process of UI, FI, and/or POP in this specialized population. Other questionnaires such as the King's Health Questionnaire and the Incontinence Impact Questionnaire have a few questions addressing sexual function but really deal with the overall impact of incontinence and/or prolapse on the patient's quality of life and well-being (Kelleher et al. 1997; Wyman et al. 1987). These questionnaires are condition-specific and were developed, validated, and tested for use in women with PFD but do not focus on sexual function. They have undergone extensive validation and reliability testing.

Other studies have shown that self-evaluation and sexual diary keeping may improve aspects of sexual life, such as couple communication, without a direct effect on variables measured with validated questionnaires on different domains of sexual function (Muin et al. 2016).

10.4   Generalized Questionnaires to Assess FSD

Questionnaires play an integral role in the evaluation of female sexual function. Although there are several questionnaires available now which deal with female sexual dysfunction, only two have a Grade A recommendation (and will be discussed in more depth), having demonstrated not only reliability and validity but also that content was derived with patient input and responsiveness to treatment has been shown.

Questionnaires available to identify or diagnose a sexual dysfunction in women include the Brief Index of Sexual Functioning for Women (Taylor et al. 1994), the short scale McCoy Female Sexuality Questionnaire (Dennerstein 2001), the Female Sexual Function Index (Rosen et al. 2000), the Changes in Sexual Functioning Questionnaire (Clayton et al. 1997), the Daily Log of Sexual Activities (Leonard et al. 2010), the Sexual Interest and Desire Inventory Female (Clayton et al. 2010), and the Multidimensional Sexuality Questionnaire (Snell Jr et al. 1993).

The Sexual Quality of Life-Female (Symonds et al. 2005) is used to assess the impact of FSD on QoL and the Sexual Function Questionnaire (Quirk et al. 2002) addresses the consequences of FSD for the woman, her partner and their relationship. It is interesting to note that the Golombok-Rust Inventory of Sexual Satisfaction (GRISS) (Rust and Golombok 1986) is the only questionnaires designed for couples to complete, not only to assess if the other partner has a sexual problem but also to assess the impact of their partner's problem on them.

Table 10.1 lists all of the questionnaires available to assess sexual function in women and reports the specific aims of each questionnaire as well as the group of patients in which they are validated. The questionnaires rating as set by the ICI is also noted

Table 10.1 Description of questionnaires to assess SF

Questionnaire name	Number of questions	Primary goal of PROM	Population Used for validation	ICI recommendation
Brief Index of Sexual Functioning in Women (BISF-W)	22	Self-administered questionnaire designed to assess current levels of female sexual functioning and satisfaction	Hetero- and homosexual women seeking routine gynaecological care with organic and inorganic causes of FSD	B
McCoy Female Sexuality Questionnaire (MFSQ)	19	Self-administered questionnaire to assess aspects of female sexual function	Postmenopausal women	C
Female Sexual Function Index (FSFI)	19	Self-administered questionnaire assessing key dimensions of sexual function in women	Normal women without any reported sexual problems and women with OAB, SUI, and MUI	A
Changes in Sexual Functioning Questionnaire- Female (CSFQ-F)	35	A gender-specific self-reported inventory designed to measure illness and medication related changes in sexual functioning (based on CSFQ structured interview design)	Medical students and patients with depression	B
Daily log of Sexual Activities	9	Self-administered questionnaire designed to provide an outcome measure of the number of sexual events, the number of satisfactory sexual events, and the magnitude of sexual interest or desire	Women with and without HSDD	B

Table 10.1 (continued)

Questionnaire name	Number of questions	Primary goal of PROM	Population Used for validation	ICI recommendation
Sexual Interest and Desire Inventory-Female (SIDI-F)	13	Clinician administered tool to quantify the severity of symptoms in women with HSDD and change in HSDD in response to treatment	Women with HSDD	B
Multidimensional Sexuality Questionnaire	12	Self-administered questionnaire designed to measure psychological tendencies associated with sexual relationships	Male and female university students	Not rated
Sexual Quality of Life-Female (SQoL-F) Questionnaire	18	Self-administered questionnaire to assess the impact of FSD on a women's sexual quality of life and to evaluate the benefits of therapeutic intervention	Women	B
Female Sexual Distress Scale-Revised (FSDS-R)	13	Self-administered questionnaire that assesses distress associated HSDD and other female sexual dysfunctions	Pre- and postmenopausal women with and without FSD	B
Derogatis Sexual Functioning Inventory (DSFI)	25	A self-reported version of semi-structured interviews designed to provide a multidimensional assessment of sexual function in men and women	Community samples of men and women—no validation in women with FSD	B
Golombok Rust Inventory of Sexual Satisfaction (GRISS)	56	A self-administered questionnaire to evaluate both the quality of a heterosexual relationship and each partner's level of sexual functioning within that relationship	Heterosexual couples from general population, gynae clinics, and sex therapy groups	A

10.5   Female Sexual Function Index (FSFI)

The FSFI was developed by a multidisciplinary group of experts in female sexual dysfunction (FSD) with question selection and domain categories based on the American Foundation for Urologic Disease classification of FSD (female sexual arousal disorder, hypoactive sexual desire disorder, female sexual orgasmic disorder, and female sexual pain disorder) (Rosen et al. 2000). The FSFI consists of a 19-item survey assessing six domains of FSD and emphasizes the domain of female sexual arousal disorder which was divided into two separate domains of lubrication and arousal to assess both the peripheral (lubrication) and central (subjective arousal and desire) components. Scores range from 2 to 36.0, with a total score of 26 or less suggestive of FSD and individual domain scores of less than 3.6 abnormal (Wiegal et al. 2005). The FSFI has been validated based on Diagnostic and Statistical Manual of Mental Disorders IV (DSM-IV) diagnoses of female sexual dysfunctions including hypoactive sexual desire disorder, female sexual arousal disorder, and female sexual orgasmic disorder (Meston 2003).

10.6   Golombok-Rust Inventory of Sexual satisfaction [GRISS]

The Golombok-Rust Inventory of Sexual Satisfaction (GRISS) is a short 28-item questionnaire for assessing the existence and severity of sexual problems. The design, construction, and item analysis of the GRISS are described. It has been shown to have high reliability and good validity for both the overall scales and the subscales. The GRISS is used by sexual dysfunction clinics and by relationship counsellors to monitor the state of their patient's sexual function. It has also been used in clinical trials of new treatment approaches and pharmacological products designed for treatment of sexual dysfunction. It is particularly useful in identifying the extent of any change in sexual function as a result of therapy. The female version of the GRISS produces a total score as well as subscales of:

- Infrequency—Number of times a week (or less) on which sexual intercourse takes place.
- Avoidance—Extent to which a female partner is actively avoiding having sex.
- Anorgasmia—Extent to which a woman is able to attain orgasm.
- Non-communication—Extent to which a couple is able to talk about any sexual problems.
- Non-sensuality—Extent to which a female partner gains pleasure from touching and caressing.
- Dissatisfaction—Extent to which a woman is dissatisfied with her sexual partner.
- Vaginismus—Extent of any tightness around the vagina that interferes with sex.

10.7   Condition-Specific Questionnaire to Assess FSD in Women with PFD

This section will specifically examine those PROMs identified by the ICI (Abrams et al. 2017) that have been validated to assess the impact of UI/POP on SF in women.

The PISQ-12 assesses sexual function after surgery in women with UI and POP (Rogers et al. 2003). The Prolapse and Incontinence Sexual Questionnaire—IUGA revised (PISQ-IR) (Rogers and Pons 2013) was developed to assess the impact of pelvic problems on sexual desire, frequency, satisfaction, orgasm, and discomfort (Abrams et al. 2017). It is the only questionnaire designed to also assess women who are not sexually active due to their condition and the impact this has on QoL and those who are sexually active without a partner. The Sexual Function Questionnaire (SFQ) is the only questionnaire specifically designed to assess SF in women with OAB (Symonds et al. 2012). Table 10.2 presents all the identified questionnaires by the ICI to assess SF in women with LUTS, reporting their primary goal and their ICI rating.

10.8   International Consultation on Incontinence Questionnaire-Vaginal Symptoms (ICIQ-VS) and International Consultation on Incontinence Questionnaire-Female Lower Urinary Tract Symptoms Sex (ICIQ-FLUTSsex)

The ICIQ-VS is a questionnaire for evaluating vaginal symptoms, associated sexual matters, and impact on quality of life (QoL) in research and clinical practice across the world. It contains 14 items and includes questions related to the respondents current sex life and worries about the effect their vagina has on their sex life and relationships.

The ICIQ-FLUTS-sex was developed to assess sexual matters associated with urinary symptoms and related bother. It consist of four items—pain/discomfort because of dry vagina, impact of urinary symptoms, pain with sexual intercourse, and urine leakage with sexual intercourse.

These ICI questionnaires are the only two with grade A recommendation and these are suggested for use in all women to measure success of treatment for PFD and are used as the outcome measures on the International Urogynaecology Associations surgical database and on many national versions around the world.

10.9   Pelvic Organ Prolapse Urinary Incontinence Sexual Questionnaire (PISQ)

The original long form of the PISQ has 31 questions and contains three domains: behavioural-emotive, physical, and partner-related. The behavioural-emotive domain measures the frequency of sexual activity, the desired frequency, orgasm

Table 10.2 Condition-specific questionnaires to assess the impact of LUTS on SF

Questionnaire name	Number of questions	Primary goal of PROM	Population Used for validation	ICI recommendation
International Consultation on Incontinence questionnaire-Vaginal symptoms (ICIQ-VS)	14	Self-administered questionnaire to assess the effects of vaginal symptoms and associated sexual matter on sexual quality of life for sexually active females	Women	A
International Consultation on Incontinence Questionnaire-Female Lower Urinary Tract Symptoms Sex (ICIQ-FLUTSsex)	4	Self-administered questionnaire to assess sexual matters associated with urinary symptoms and related bother		A
Pelvic Organ Prolapse/Urinary Incontinence Sexual Questionnaire (PISQ)	31	To assess sexual function after surgery in women with pelvic floor dysfunction	Women with pelvic floor dysfunction	B
Pelvic Organ Prolapse/Urinary Incontinence Sexual Questionnaire short form (PISQ-12)	12	To assess sexual function in women with incontinence and prolapse	Women with pelvic floor dysfunction	B
Pelvic Organ Prolapse/Urinary Incontinence Sexual Questionnaire IUGA revised (PISQ-IR)	19	Self-administered questionnaire assessing key dimensions of sexual function including bother in women who are sexually active and those who do not report sexual activity		C
Sexual Function Questionnaire	31	Self-administered questionnaire used to assess the impact of OAB on sexual health/function in the male and female population	Men and women with OAB	C

rates, and satisfaction with one's sexual relationship. The physical domain examines episodes of pain, incontinence, sensation of prolapse, and fear of faecal and/or urinary incontinence during sexual activity. The partner-related domain includes any difficulty with erectile dysfunction, premature ejaculation, vaginal attenuation, vaginal tightness, or the patient's perception of a partner's avoidance of intercourse.

The PISQ has undergone criterion or construct validity and external validation. Additionally, the PISQ is able to distinguish between women with and without high depression scores on the symptom questionnaire, with depression associated with, and an alternative of, poor sexual function. The PISQ utilizes a Likert scale with 0 = never and 4 = always, with reverse scoring used on some questions to consistently reflect that higher scores equal better sexual function with a maximal score of 124 possible. Normative scores were not established in the original questionnaire development, but the mean score in a healthy population used to validate the questionnaire was 94 (Rogers et al. 2001). A short form of the PISQ has also been validated and contains 12 questions (PISQ-12) (Rogers et al. 2003). The PISQ-12 has a maximal score of 48 and can be converted to PISQ Long Form scores when multiplied by 2.58.

The PISQ has also been validated Portuguese and Spanish, both in America and Spain (Pons et al. 2008; Romero et al. 2003). A Medline search noted 27 publications utilizing the PISQ not including abstracts or other citations, furthering the validation process. The PISQ was recently utilized in a general population of twins to evaluate for sexual dysfunction and establish normative values (Aschkenzi et al. 2008). The PISQ-12 scores highly correlated with scores of a general sexual function questionnaire and were significantly lower in women with depressive symptoms or pain of bladder origin. These findings suggest that PISQ-12 may be reliably used in a general population without PFD. The mean PISQ-12 score in their population of sexually active women without bothersome POP or UI was 40. The short form has been proven to demonstrate excellent correlation with the full version but reduces time and burden on the patients who are completing the questionnaire (Rogers et al. 2003). A lower score represents better SF.

10.10 The Impact of Pelvic Floor Dysfunction on Sexual Function

The effect of PFD on sexual function has been evaluated using validated quality-of-life PFD dysfunction and sexual function questionnaires. Handa et al. (2008) utilized the Pelvic Floor Disorders Inventory 20 (PFDI-20) as well as the Personal Experience Questionnaire, a non-condition-specific validated generalized sexual function questionnaire, and found that higher PFDI-20 scores were associated with decreased arousal, infrequent orgasm, and increased dyspareunia, with similar findings noted for the urinary, colorectal-anal, and prolapse scales of the PFDI-20 (Handa et al. 2008). The only sexual problem associated with increasing prolapse was infrequent orgasm. A recent community-based survey assessed the relationship between PFD and sexual activity and satisfaction using the Epidemiology of Prolapse and Incontinence Questionnaire (EPIQ) (Lukacz et al. 2007). The EPIQ was specifically designed to ascertain the prevalence of and risk factors for PFD in an undiagnosed population and includes questions that are related specifically to sexual activity and satisfaction. After controlling for confounding variables, PFD was not significantly associated with sexual activity or satisfaction, but only 43% of the women who had PFD based on EPIQ had sought care for their conditions.

10.11 Effects of Gynaecologic Surgeries on Sexual Function

The effects of gynaecologic surgery on sexual function have historically received little attention. Due to the use of different and mainly non-validated, self-made questionnaires, lack of definition of sexual function and dysfunction, and non-assessment of impact on QOL, it is difficult to compare older studies and draw conclusions. A recent comprehensive review of the literature found 36 articles involving 4500 patients, and only 12 used validated questionnaires to assess sexual function after surgery for PFD (Ghielmetti et al. 2006). Conflicting results were noted with some studies suggesting that surgery for POP and UI deteriorates sexual function, some demonstrating no change and others, improvement in sexual function. The authors concluded that there was a 'paucity of properly validated data about sexual function after gynaecologic operations' and urged further prospective studies using validated questionnaires. Since this publication, there have been several more well-designed studies assessing the outcomes of surgery for PFD with respect to sexual function.

The PISQ-12 has also been used to prospectively evaluate sexual function after surgical treatment for PFD. The other questionnaire utilized to assess sexual function after surgical treatment of PFD is the FSFI, which is validated, but generalized or non-condition-specific. Many recent publications examining the impact of UI, FI, and POP using the FSFI and PISQ have reported poorer sexual function in women with PFD. The PISQ has been used most commonly to evaluate sexual function after surgery for PFD, with increased PISQ scores in about 70%. Significant improvement is noted for sexual function related to physical and partner-related factors, with no changes for orgasm, desire, or arousal after surgical repair of PFD. Studies which used generalized sexual function questionnaires mostly found no change in sexual function following surgical treatment of POP and/or UI. When evaluated with validated questionnaires, PFD is associated with a negative impact on sexual function. Surgical correction of POP and/or UI improves sexual function in about 70%, although some studies show no change with the use of non-condition-specific questionnaires.

10.12 Conclusion

Sexual dysfunction is often complex and biopsychosocial. It involves a complex interplay of biological, psychological, interpersonal, and sociocultural factors. A multidisciplinary clinic is uniquely equipped to address sexual health problems. Identification of sexual health concerns engages diagnostic components of psychologic consultation, history, physical examination, and laboratory testing as appropriate. The use of subjective and objective outcome measures enables the assessment and re-evaluation of symptoms and their impact on quality of life to be measured in a valid and reliable way. This can not only inform treatment success in the individual but allow comparisons of outcomes across locations and differing interventions.

References

Abrams P, Cardozo L, Wein A, Wagg A (eds) (2017) Incontinence, 6th edn. Health Publications Ltd, Cork

Althof SE, Symonds T (2007) Patient reported outcomes used in the assessment of premature ejaculation. Urol Clin North Am 34:581–589

Aschkenzi SO, Botros SM, Beaumont J, Miller JJ, Gamble T, Sand PK, Goldberg RP (2008) Use of the short pelvic organ prolapse/urinary incontinence sexual questionnaire for female sexual dysfunction in a general population. Obstet Gynecol 111(4S):10S

Clayton AH, McGarvey EL, Clavet GJ (1997) The Changes in Sexual Functioning Questionnaire (CSFQ): development, reliability, and validity. Psychopharmacol Bull 33(4):731

Clayton AH, Goldmeier D, Nappi RE, Wunderlich G, Lewis-D'Agostino DJ, Pyke R (2010) Validation of the sexual interest and desire inventory-female in hypoactive sexual desire disorder. J Sex Med 7(12):3918–3928

Dennerstein L, Lehert P, Dudley E (2001) Short scale to measure female sexuality: adapted from McCoy Female Sexuality Questionnaire. J Sex Marital Ther 27(4):339–351

Ghielmetti T, Kuhn P, Dreher EF, Kuhn A (2006) Gynaecological operations: do they improve sexual life? Eur J Obstet Gynecol Reprod Biol 129:104–110

Handa VL, Cundif G, Chang HH, Helzlsouer KJ (2008) Female sexual function and pelvic floor disorders. Obstet Gynecol 111:1045–1052

Kelleher CJ, Cardozo LD, Khullar V, Salvatore S (1997) A new questionnaire to assess the quality of life of urinary incontinent women. BJOG Int J Obstet Gynaecol 104(12):1374–1379

Leonard R, DeRogatis LR, Allgood A, Auerbach P, Eubank D, Greist J, Bharmal M, Zipfel L, Guo CY (2010) Validation of a women's sexual interest diagnostic interview—short form (WSID-SF) and a daily log of sexual activities (DLSA) in postmenopausal women with hypoactive sexual desire disorder. J Sex Med 7(2 pt 2):917–927

Lukacz ES, Whitcomb EL, Lawrence JM, Nager CW, Contreras R, Luber KM (2007) Are sexual activity and satisfaction affected by pelvic floor disorders? Analysis of a community-based survey. Am J Obstet Gynecol 197:e1–88.e6

Meston CM (2003) Validation of the Female Sexual Function Index (FSFI) in women with female orgasmic disorder and in women with hypoactive sexual desire disorder. J Sex Marital Ther 29:39–46

Muin DA, Wolzt M, Rezaei SS, Tremmel-Scheinost M, Salama M, Fuchs C, Luger A, Müller M, Bayerle-Eder M (2016) Effect of sexual diary keeping and self-evaluation on female sexual function and depression: a pilot study. Eur J Contracept Reprod Health Care 21(2):141–149

Pauls RN, Segal JL, Silva WA, Kleeman SD, Karram MM (2006) Sexual function in patients presenting to a urogynecology practice. Int Urogynecol J Pelvic Floor Dysfunct 17(6):576–580

Pons EM, Clota PM, Aguilon GM, Zardain PC, Alvarez RP (2008) Questionnaire for evaluation of sexual function in women with genital prolapse and/or incontinence. Validation of the Spanish version of "Pelvic Organ Prolapse/Urinary Incontinence Sexual Questionnaire (PISQ-12)". Actas Urol Esp 32:211–219

Quirk FH, Heiman JR, Rosen RC, Laan E, Smith MD, Boolell M (2002) Development of a sexual function questionnaire for clinical trials of female sexual dysfunction. J Womens Health Gend Based Med 11(3):277–289

Rogers RG, Pons ME (2013) The pelvic organ prolapse incontinence sexual questionnaire, IUGA-revised (PISQ-IR)

Rogers RG, Villarreal A, Kammerer-Doak D, Qualls C (2001) Sexual function in women with and without urinary incontinence and/or pelvic organ prolapse. Int Urogynecol J Pelvic Floor Dysfunct 12(6):361–365

Rogers RG, Coates KW, Kammerer-Doak D, Khalsa S, Qualls C (2003) A short form of the pelvic organ prolapse/urinary incontinence sexual questionnaire (PISQ-12). Int Urogynecol J 14(3):164–168

Rogers RG, Rockwood TH, Constantine ML, Thakar R, Kammerer-Doak DN, Pauls RN, Parekh M, Ridgeway B, Jha S, Pitkin J, Reid F (2013) A new measure of sexual function in women with pelvic floor disorders (PFD): the Pelvic Organ Prolapse/Incontinence Sexual Questionnaire, IUGA-Revised (PISQ-IR). Int Urogynecol J 24(7):1091–1103

Romero AA, Hardart A, Rogers R, Kobak B (2003) Validation of a Spanish version of the Pelvic Organ Prolapse Incontinence Sexual Questionnaire (PISQ). Obstet Gynecol 102:1000–1005

Rosen C, Brown J, Heiman S, Leiblum C, Meston R, Shabsigh D, Ferguson R, D'Agostino R (2000) The Female Sexual Function Index (FSFI): a multidimensional self-report instrument for the assessment of female sexual function. J Sex Marital Ther 26(2):191–208

Rust J, Golombok S (1986) The GRISS: a psychometric instrument for the assessment of sexual dysfunction. Arch Sex Behav 15(2):157–165

Snell WE Jr, Fisher TD, Walters AS (1993) The Multidimensional Sexuality Questionnaire: an objective self-report measure of psychological tendencies associated with human sexuality. Ann Sex Res 6(1):27–55

Symonds T, Boolell M, Quirk F (2005) Development of a questionnaire on sexual quality of life in women. J Sex Marital Ther 31(5):385–397

Symonds T, Abraham L, Bushmakin AG, Williams K, Martin M, Cappelleri JC (2012) Sexual function questionnaire: further refinement and validation. J Sex Med 9(10):2609–2616

Taylor JF, Rosen RC, Leiblum SR (1994) Self-report assessment of female sexual function: psychometric evaluation of the Brief Index of Sexual Functioning for Women. Arch Sex Behav 23(6):627–643

Temml C, Haidinger G, Schmidbauer J, Schatzl G, Madersbacher S (2000) Urinary incontinence in both sexes: prevalence rates and impact on quality of life and sexual life. Neurourol Urodyn 19:259–271

WHO (2006) Defining sexual health: report of a technical consultation on sexual health, 28–31 January 2002. World Health Organization, Geneva

Wiegal M, Meston C, Rosen R (2005) The Female Sexual Function Index (FSFI): cross-validation and development of clinical cutoff scores. J Sex Marital Ther 31:1–20

Wyman JF, Harkins SW, Choi SC, Taylor JR, Fantl JA (1987) Psychosocial impact of urinary incontinence in women. Obstet Gynecol 70:378–381

Over the Counter and Home Remedies

11

Ellie Stewart

11.1 Vaginal Dryness

Vaginal dryness can affect women of any age and can be multifaceted. There are a number of causes and symptoms of vaginal dryness (detailed in Tables 11.1 and 11.2) and often something as simple as an effective, appropriate lubrication can be enough to improve symptoms.

Vaginal dryness is common symptom of the menopause (Edwards and Panay 2015a). It can affect over half of post-menopausal women aged between 51 and 60. Vaginal tissues are oestrogen dependent, so as oestrogen levels drop during and

Table 11.1 Causes of vaginal dryness

Causes of vaginal dryness
Giving birth and breastfeeding
Medications—antidepressants, antihistamines
Perfumed soaps, vaginal douches
Hormone replacement therapy (HRT) and contraception such as the coil and pill
Menopause

Table 11.2 Symptoms of vaginal dryness

Symptoms of vaginal dryness
Dyspareunia
Dryness
Stinging, burning, swelling
Vulval discomfort
Bleeding

E. Stewart (✉)
Gynaecology, West Suffolk Hospital NHS Foundation Trust, Suffolk, UK
e-mail: Ellie.Stewart@wsh.nhs.uk

© Springer Nature Switzerland AG 2021
A. Rantell (ed.), *Sexual Function and Pelvic Floor Dysfunction*,
https://doi.org/10.1007/978-3-030-63843-6_11

after the menopause, the vagina can become dry and the tissues become thinner, more fragile and sensitive. Women often find that they don't lubricate sufficiently for sex to be comfortable after the menopause (Edwards and Panay 2015a). They may feel turned on mentally, but the vagina doesn't lubricate adequately to allow for comfortable penetration.

Women may try an additional lubrication or moisturisers to reduce the discomfort. There are a number of lubricants available for women to purchase and many women will have tried a few of these in an attempt to reduce the dryness and discomfort and allow for comfortable love making before seeking help.

11.2 Lubrication

Lubrications can be bought over the counter in pharmacies, chemists, supermarkets and online. There has been a recent increase in the number of lubrications available to purchase. Women no longer opt for the traditional KY jelly, which can dry out the vagina when used during sexual intercourse, and are moving to lubrications with flavour, or a tingle or ones which are oil/water based. And with women wanting to avoid seeing a healthcare professional to discuss problems which they consider to be embarrassing, the advent of support groups available on social media and a cohort of younger women discussing their vaginal health more readily, women are likely to have tried them before seeking help.

There are two main types of vaginal lubrication.

11.2.1 Water-Based Lubrication

Water-based lubricants are the most common lubricants available. They come in two varieties: with glycerin or without glycerin. Both types of water-based lubricant are cost-effective, easy to find in the shops or online and are safe to use with condoms. They usually don't stain the sheets which is an important consideration. Glycerin-free products are less likely to cause vaginal irritation. They also have a longer shelf life.

11.2.2 Oil-Based Lubrication

Oil-based lubes are often sticky, greasy and can corrode latex condoms and diaphragms. Oil-based lubricants are commonly used because they are often readily available around the house—some of these include Vaseline, baby oil, mineral oil and even cooking oils. But there are also a number of different ones to purchase online.

11.2.3 Vaginal Moisturisers

Some women may have tried using vaginal moisturisers as an alternative to vaginal oestrogen, as this currently can't be bought over the counter, when experiencing a sore, dry, uncomfortable vagina. Vaginal moisturisers moisturise the vagina by attaching onto the dry walls of the vagina, thereby mimicking natural vaginal secretions (Edwards and Panay 2015b), where needed, rehydrating the dry mucosa. They are often pH matched to help restore and maintain vaginal health and are latex/condom friendly. They need to be reapplied every 3 days.

11.2.4 Topical Vaginal Oestrogens

These aren't available over the counter but can be prescribed by a healthcare professional if vaginal dryness remains a problem so these won't have been tried prior to seeing a healthcare professional.

11.3 Dyspareunia

Some women suffer significantly with painful sex. This may be attributed to a number of factors/conditions such as pelvic pain, prolapse, menopause, endometriosis, post childbirth, vaginismus and vulvodynia.

Women experiencing dyspareunia due to yeast or urinary tract infections often self-medicate with clotrimazole pessaries and creams or an anti-cystitis remedy. Once the infection is treated, the dyspareunia should go.

Some more complex causes of dyspareunia such as vulvodynia, vaginismus and endometriosis can be difficult to manage. Women will try and manage these symptoms and conditions at home, often for long periods of time, before discussing with their healthcare professional. They will head to the internet and social media groups for support and ideas for managing their conditions.

Below are some of the things that women may have tried to enable a normal sexual relationship:

11.3.1 Dyspareunia Due to Vaginal Dryness

Some women may be put off having sex due to the discomfort felt as a result of their dry vagina. Some women experience vaginal dryness during sex because they are not sufficiently sexually aroused. This may be due to psychological reasons, such as stress and anxiety, or tiredness, chronic pain conditions and depression. Some womens vaginas become dry around the menopause, but vaginal dryness can also be caused by a lack of/insufficient foreplay. Women will often try to spice up their love lives by cooking a nice romantic meal for their partner, wearing sexy underwear, dressing up or trying some erotic literature.

Vaginal dryness can also be linked to overuse of perfumed soaps, bubble baths, feminine washes and wipes or over-douching. These things are readily available to buy, but women are often unaware of the effects on their vagina. They should be advised to avoid overwashing their vagina and to use a natural soap such as dove or simple, to try and reduce any dryness. Overwashing can strip the vagina of its natural flora and change its pH which in turn can cause irritation and infections such as candida (quote) and bacterial vaginosis.

11.3.2 Vulvodynia

Women may have tried anti-inflammatory medications to try and help manage the pain that they are experiencing in their vulva. They may also have tried cognitive behavioural therapy (CBT) or some form of sexual therapy. Couples may have also approached a psychosexual counsellor for advice on how to manage their sexual issues and concerns. A diet low in oxalate salts may have been tried as a treatment for women who experience vulval pain or vulvodynia. A diet low in oxalate with or without calcium citrate may benefit some women with vulval pain (http://www. vulvalpainsociety.org/vps/index.php/treatments/the-low-oxalate-diet. Accessed 23 Nov 2019). Oxalate is a chemical found in plant foods. Table 11.3 details examples of foods to avoid when eating a low oxalate diet. Some women may have tried bathing the vulva once or twice a day with compresses soaked in colloidal oatmeal which has previously been dissolved in water, or by sitting in a bath with colloidal oatmeal product in it.

Table 11.3 Foods to avoid in a low oxalate diet

Grains
Wheat bran, wheat germ and barley
Grits and bran cereal
White corn flour and buckwheat flour
Whole wheat bread
Vegetables
Collard greens, leeks, okra and spinach
Wax beans
Eggplant
Beets and beet greens
Swiss chard, escarole, parsley and rutabagas
Tomato paste
Protein foods
Baked beans with tomato sauce
Nut butters and nuts (peanuts, almonds, hazelnuts)
Soy burgers
Miso
Dried beans

11.3.3 Endometriosis

Not everyone with endometriosis experiences dyspareunia, but of those who do some will experience pain after sex and others during sex or deep penetrative sex (https://www.endometriosis-uk.org/endometriosis-and-couples. Accessed 2 Dec 2019). This can range from mild to severe in severity.

Women may have tried a number of different sexual positions to help with the dyspareunia as some may not cause as much pain or discomfort. For example, when the person with endometriosis is on top they can control the depth and speed of penetration allowing them to determine a pace which is comfortable for them. Some other positions women may have tried are modified doggy style, spooning, raising the hips of the person with endometriosis in the missionary position.

Sometimes any form of penetrative sex is painful and the couple may prefer to engage in other types of sexual activity. Women may have tried other things such as oral sex, massage, extended foreplay and toys.

The ohnut (https://ohnut.co/blogs/journal. Accessed 13 Nov 2019) allows for penetration, but at the depth which is comfortable and tolerated. Each set comes with four linking rings which allow for differing levels of penetration depending on comfort. It is placed over the erect penis and intercourse is attempted. This may suit women with endometriosis who have collision dyspareunia (previously known as deep dyspareunia).

11.3.4 Post Brachytherapy

Brachytherapy for treatment of cervical and endometrial cancer can cause problems with vaginal stenosis. Women often suffer with problems with penetration and sore fragile vaginal tissues. Often women who have been treated with brachytherapy will have tried vaginal dilators with the hope of gaining vaginal function again. They may also have tried vaginal lubrications and moisturisers to aid sexual contact.

11.4   Incontinence

Urinary incontinence is a very common problem experienced by women of all ages (Stewart 2019). The EPIC study (Coyne et al. 2009) found that 66.6% of women over the age of 40 years suffered with at least one lower urinary tract symptom. Women, as copers, will often have tried a number of different strategies to help manage or contain their symptoms before seeking help. Stopping smoking can help to reduce coughing. Women with chronic coughs can suffer with urinary leakage or pelvic floor dysfunction due to the raise in intraabdominal pressure with each cough. There are government schemes which women can enrol on to help and support them to stop smoking. Women with constipation who strain to open their bowels can help improve their pelvic floor symptoms (leakage and prolapse) by regulating their bowels and avoiding straining.

Some of the other strategies women may have tried to improve their urinary incontinence are detailed below.

11.4.1 Pelvic Floor Exercises

Women are likely to have tried some sort of pelvic floor exercises before seeking help. There are many websites available which describe how to do these exercises correctly, or some women may have been taught how to do them via word of mouth—from their mum or friend.

There are a number of apps, some of which are free and some paid for, which remind women to do their exercises regularly—for example the squeezy app (https://www.squeezyapp.com). Women may find information about these online or after speaking to their peers.

There are a number of vaginal devices available online, which women may have found when searching around the topic and tried prior to referral. Vaginal cones can be inserted into the vagina and as the pelvic floor strengthens, the weights inserted inside the cone can be increased, which in turn makes the muscle work harder and improve its strength.

Electrical stimulation machines may have been tried before seeking help. These are available online. These can be bought for as little as £50 or women can pay significantly more for them.

Intravaginal feedback devices can be purchased and used. These are inserted into the vagina and synched to the mobile phone. When the pelvic floor is squeezed, a biofeedback mechanism is activated, so the woman using it can see how hard they are squeezing their muscle, can refine their technique if they aren't doing it correctly and can see how their muscle strength is improving.

Sometimes using these machines, devices or apps can mean that that their symptoms improve significantly enough for them not to need to see their GP for referral to secondary care.

11.4.2 Intravaginal Support Devices

Intravaginal devices are available to purchase, they aim to support the bladder neck and prevent symptoms of stress urinary incontinence. The devices sit inside the vagina and support the bladder neck (Fig. 11.1), so when there is a raise in intraabdominal pressure the leakage is reduced, or stops. Some of the in devices available in the UK are pictured below in Figs. 11.2, 11.3, 11.4 and 11.5. Some women may have tried using a tampon in their vagina whilst exercising to help reduce urinary leakage as they were unaware of the devices available.

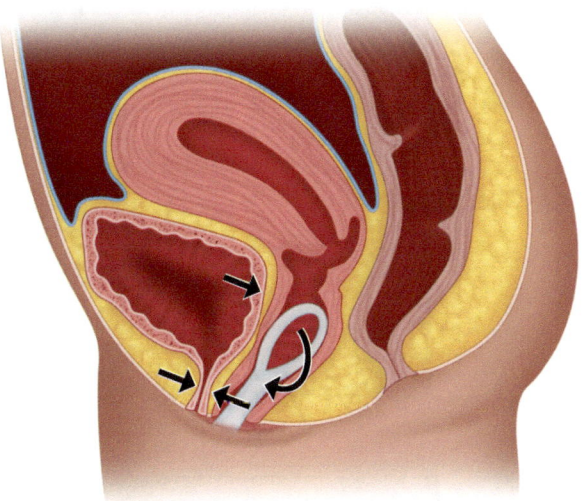

Fig. 11.1 Correct position of device in vagina. With permission from BBraun

Fig. 11.2 Diveen

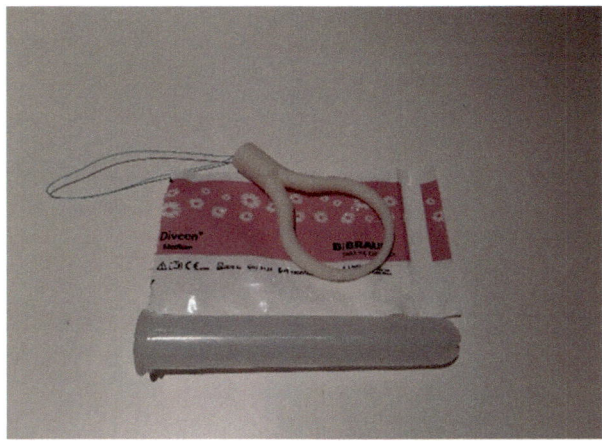

Fig. 11.3 Uresta

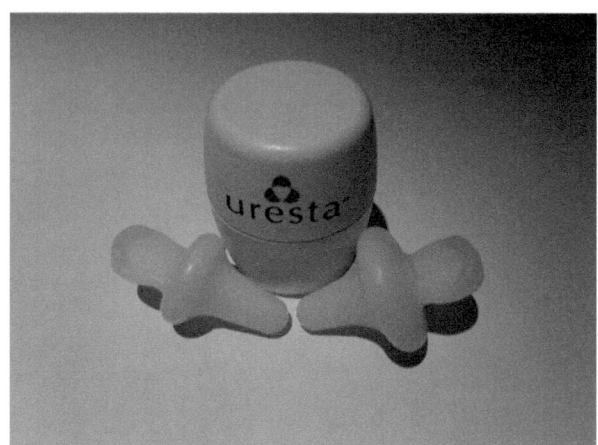

Fig. 11.4 Aquaflex cones

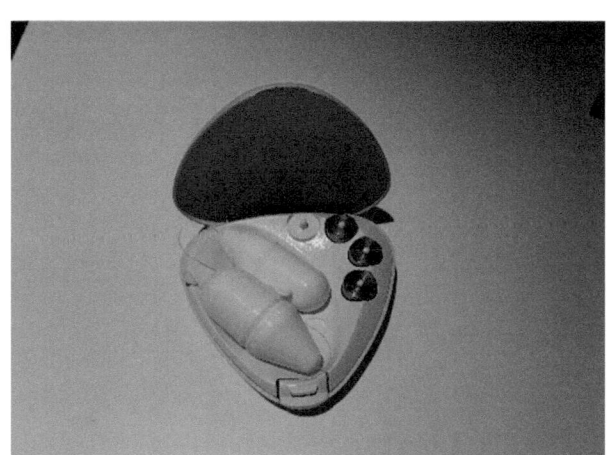

Fig. 11.5 Contiform

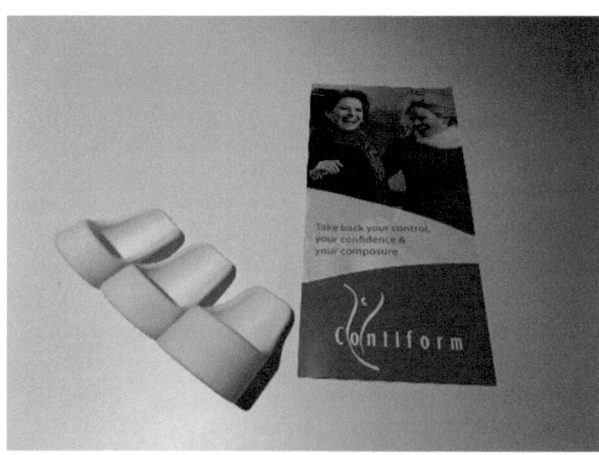

Table 11.4 Simple strategies for reducing leakage during sex

Avoiding foods or drinks which may irritate the bladder a couple of hours before sex
Using protective bedding
Going to the toilet before sex to reduce leakage
Having sex in the shower
Discussing concerns with a partner—who may be willing to try different positions/non-penetrative sex

These intravaginal devices can be purchased online, can significantly improve symptoms and can be a useful adjunct for women working on their pelvic floor exercises (Al-Shaikh et al. 2018). Women who chose to use these devices may notice an improvement in their symptoms during the day but it is important to note that they can't be worn during sex (Fig. 11.5).

Women may have been put off surgery following the recent mesh scandal and mesh suspension—so they may have turned to the internet to suggest other ways of managing their symptoms.

11.4.3 Weight Loss

Obesity is a significant, adjustable and reversible risk factor for stress incontinence (Faiena et al. 2015). Subak et al. (2009) suggest that moderate weight loss may decrease episodes of urinary incontinence. Women may have tried weight loss as a way of trying to boost their self-confidence and improve their image or purely to see if it would improve their symptoms. Women may have tried self-help groups such as weight watchers or slimming world, or may have tried dieting at home.

11.4.4 Sexual Positions

Women may have tried some simple strategies to reduce urinary leakage during sex—see Table 11.4. Changing the position you have sex in can reduce urinary leakage. Some women suggest that the missionary position and doggy style can press on the bladder and irritate it, which in turn may cause incontinence. Instead, pillows can be put under the pelvis which repositions the bladder and reduces any extra pressure.

11.5 Prolapse

Pelvic organ prolapse is one of the most common medical disorders, with one in two parous women suffering with pelvic organ prolapse (POP). NHS UK (www.nhs.uk/conditions/pelvic-organ-prolapse/. Accessed 30 Nov 2019) has described a vaginal prolapse as when 'one or more of the organs in the pelvic slip down from their normal position and bulge in the vagina'. Having a vaginal prolapse may affect a woman's life in a number of ways, so by the time she presents at the GP, she is likely to have tried a number of coping strategies.

11.5.1 Sea Sponges

These are often tried by women who find that their prolapse means that they can't comfortably hold a tampon in their vagina at the time of their period. Some are unable to tolerate one at all. Sea sponges are bought online and can be cut to size. They are comfortable, non-irritating and environmentally friendly (https://menstrualcupreviews.net/sea-sponge-menstrual-soft-tampons-product-reviews/. Accessed 9 Dec 2019). They are inserted into the vagina and can be worn for up to 4 h before removing and washing and reinserting. Some women prefer using the sea sponges instead of relying on pads. These shouldn't be worn during sex.

11.5.2 Sexual Positions

Sex may become more difficult or uncomfortable with a vaginal prolapse (www.peri-coach.com/2017/20/comfortable-sex-positions-for-women-with-pelvic-floor-disorders/. Accessed 30 Nov 2019). Women may have spent time trying different sexual positions to see what is most comfortable for them and their partners. The cowgirl (woman on top) and sex standing up means that the prolapse falls down into the vagina which can make sex painful or uncomfortable (www.nafc.org/bhealth-blog/the-best-sex-positions-if-you-have-incontinence-or-pelvic-organ-prolapse. Accessed 30 Nov 2019). Instead, women may have tried the modified missionary position (where pillows are placed under the pelvis to tilt the pelvic back and allow the prolapse to move back in the vagina). Some women report that doggy style or spooning (where the man enters from behind) can temporarily improve the symptoms of a rectocele.

Often male partners are worried about having sex when their partner has a vaginal prolapse. They are worried that they may hurt them or make them worse. In some instances, they may even feel turned off by the prolapse. These scenarios can cause issues within the relationship which may be difficult to broach or discuss with a healthcare professional. For those with significant, deeper relationship issues, couples may have spoken to a counsellor or had some sort of relationship counselling.

11.5.3 Internet and Chat Rooms

Women often resort to chat rooms on the internet to discuss their problems and symptoms. They may find it easier to discuss their symptoms with the protection of anonymity, but also with women who are suffering with similar symptoms and problems.

11.5.4 Support Devices

The v-brace by fembrace is said to provide non-invasive perineal support for women with a vaginal prolapse. It lifts and supports the crotch and perineal area which may reduce symptoms.

Support shorts/underwear are also available. These provide upward compression by supporting the pelvic floor. Some women may have tried wearing tighter underwear, or wearing a couple of pads to support their perineum and find that their symptoms are improved as a result.

Women may also have tried to lose some weight and pelvic floor exercises—both of these have been discussed previously in the chapter. Weight loss may help improve a woman's sex life, but the support devices will only help with day to day management of symptoms.

11.6 Low Libido

Low libido is one of the sexual problems most commonly associated with pelvic floor dysfunction (Jha and Gopinath 2016). It is multifaceted and is often difficult to pin down to one cause. Sexual desire often decreases following childbirth, the menopause, with weight gain, depression and anxiety and how the woman feels about herself at any specific time. A reduction in libido can put strain on a relationship without any additional symptoms of pelvic floor dysfunction—such as urinary incontinence, prolapse or vaginal dryness. Women are resourceful and may have tried a number of things to increase her libido, these may include:

11.6.1 Food

Little evidence supports the effectiveness of certain foods in increasing the libido—but many women may have tried supplements or different food groups to see if they will improve symptoms. Below are a few foods which women may have tried to boost their libido.

Afoakwa (2008) has suggested that eating chocolate promotes the release of serotonin and phenylethylamine into the body which can produce some mood lifting effects. Salonia et al. (2006) however, suggests that the benefits of eating chocolate are more psychological than biological. Women may have tried eating oysters or drinking a glass of wine to help them relax which may increase their interest in sex.

Garlic has high levels of allicin which can increase blood flow and the smell of basil is known to stimulate the senses so may be used to try and increase sexual desire.

Strawberries and raspberries—these have high levels of zinc which is needed for women bodies to prepare for sex.

Watermelon—increases libido.

Avocados contain folic acid and vitamin B6 which are both necessary for a healthy sex drive. Folic acid pumps the body with energy, whilst vitamin B6 stabilises the hormones.

11.6.2 Essential Oils

Women may have tried to combine massage with libido boosting essential oils to increase their sex drive. Table 11.5 details some commonly used essential oils.

Table 11.5 Commonly used essential oils

Ylan ylan—is a natural sedative which supports a feeling of deeper connection
Ginger—gets the blood flowing and can help with building physical confidence
Rose—aids depression and stress
Clary sage—stimulating, euphoric and generally uplifting, boosts libido

11.6.3 Sex Toys and Other Erotica

Women may have chosen to spice up their sex lives with the use of sex toys, vibrators, sexy underwear and erotic literature—such as the 50 shades of grey trilogy. There has been a rise in home delivery services for sex toys and erotica. The internet has enabled women to search online for this type of product and buy them anonymously. Women may choose to order online rather than visit a shop for convenience sake, especially if their purchases are delivered in plain packaging with a discreet service.

Women may also have watched porn to try and 'spice up' their sex lives. This is much more readily available on the internet and accessible 24 h a day on mobile devices. No longer do people have to access this by buying a magazine over the counter. There are a number of porn websites available with porn categories accounting for all tastes.

11.7 Lack of Research

There is a significant lack of research available for things which women may have tried before seeking professional help for their symptoms of pelvic floor dysfunction. I performed a number of literature searches with more experienced librarians and found little, if any research. This could be because women don't want to talk about things they have tried to improve their symptoms, that people undertaking research don't feel that there is a need to look into this area or that there isn't the funding available to do so.

11.8 Women and the Internet

Women today often have easier access to the internet, and with that comes the ability to look at symptoms or a problem and find solutions. This provides information—both good and bad—for women who are seeking help for a specific problem, pelvic floor dysfunction included. Table 11.6 details some of the support groups available online to women.

Women in the twenty-first century are talking about things more readily and are less likely to 'put up' with symptoms that previous generations considered a part of

Table 11.6 Types of online support available	Blogs
	Support groups online
	Charity support groups
	Discussion and support forums, i.e. mumsnet
	Facebook groups
	Twitter groups and handles

normal ageing or something to be expected. We are more likely to ask questions and want answers, and with the internet, women can often find these answers.

11.8.1 Other Ways of Getting Information

Woman's hour on BBC radio 2 provides women with discussion and topics relevant to many health conditions. Traditional women's magazines may also discuss subjects which women don't feel they are able to approach their GP about, whether this is in an agony aunt type discussion or factual information. Popular daytime TV programmes such as 'This Morning' often have sections dedicated to showing new devices or ways of managing a specific problem. For women who don't have access to the internet, these other mediums may be ways that women obtain information.

Advertising has become more liberal. Women now see adverts for incontinence pads and vaginal moisturisers on the television and in women's magazines. Women's health is being discussed more openly on popular daytime television programmes— and women are more likely to look at the resources that these programmes suggest.

11.9   Conclusions

Women are less likely to accept that prolapse, incontinence, a dry vagina and many other symptoms of pelvic floor dysfunction are to be 'put up with' anymore and are likely to have asked friends, family or work colleagues or gone onto the internet for advice. This means that before seeking help, many women will have tried a number of self-help strategies to improve these symptoms. It is important for healthcare professionals seeing women with pelvic floor dysfunction to be aware of what they may have tried, and be able to suggest some of the less invasive options should they deem them appropriate.

References

Afoakwa E (2008) Cocoa and chocolate consumption- are there aphrodisiac and other benefits for human health? https://works.bepress.com/emmanueloheneafoakwa/90/. Accessed 27 Nov 2019

Al-Shaikh G, Syed S, Bogis A et al (2018) Pessary use in stress urinary incontinence: a review of advantages, complications, patient satisfaction and quality of life. Int J Women Health 10:195–201. https://www.ncbi.nlm.nih.gov/pmc/articles/PMC5909791/pdf/ijwh-10-195.pdf

Coyne K, Sexton C, Thompson C, Milsom I et al (2009) The prevalence of lower urinary tract symptoms (LUTS) in the USA, the UK and Sweden; results from the epidemiology of LUTs (EpiLUTS) study. Br J Urol Int 104:352–360

Edwards D, Panay N (2015a) Treating vulvovaginal atrophy/ genitourinary syndrome of menopause: how important is lubricant and moisturiser composition? Climacteric 19(2):151–161. https://doi.org/10.3109/13697137.2015.1124259

Edwards D, Panay N (2015b) Treating vulvovaginal atrophy/genitourinary syndrome of menopause: how important is vaginal lubricant and moisturizer composition? Climacteric 19(2) https://www.tandfonline.com/doi/full/10.3109/13697137.2015.1124259

Faiena I, Patel N, Parihar JS et al (2015) Conservative management of urinary incontinence in women. Rev Urol 17(3):129–139

Jha S, Gopinath D (2016) Prolapse or incontinence: what affects sexual function the most? Int Urogynaecol J 27:607–611

Salonia A, Fabbin F et al (2006) Original research—womens sexual health: chocolate and womens sexual health: an intriguing correlation. J Sex Med 3(3):476–482. https://doi.org/10.1111/j.1743-6109.2006.00236.x

Stewart E (2019) Urogynaecology. In: Nursing management of women's health: guide for nurse specialists and practitioners. Springer, New York, NY, pp 215–234

Subak LL, Wing R, Smith West DS et al (2009) Weight loss to treat urinary incontinence in overweight and obsess women. N England J Med 360(5):481–491

Psychosexual Therapy for Female Sexual Dysfunction (FSD)

12

Angela Gregory

Key Points
- Sexual functioning is a quality of life issue.
- Clinicians have an important role in the early detection of sexual problems.
- Early intervention can prevent more complex problems from developing.
- A multi-disciplinary approach often provides the best outcome for women with sexual difficulties.
- Psychosexual therapy can be beneficial for women experiencing sexual difficulities.

12.1 Introduction

12.1.1 Psychosexual Therapy

Historically, psychosexual therapy was a specialised form of cognitive behavioural psychotherapy that explored, challenged and reframed detrimental cognitions and utilised specific behavioural strategies carried out by individuals and couples in their home environment. The behavioural aspect of this treatment approach is often referred to as 'Sensate Focus' (Masters and Johnson 1970). However, contemporary psychosexual therapy may also include an array of other technical interventions known to effectively treat sexual difficulties such as systems/couple interventions and sometimes psychodynamic/psychoanalytic interventions (Kirana 2013a). Ideally these should be combined with a medical assessment and pharmacological therapy if

A. Gregory (✉)
Department of Sexual Health, Chandos Clinic, Nottingham University Hospital Trust, Nottingham, UK
e-mail: Angela.Gregory@nuh.nhs.uk

© Springer Nature Switzerland AG 2021
A. Rantell (ed.), *Sexual Function and Pelvic Floor Dysfunction*,
https://doi.org/10.1007/978-3-030-63843-6_12

137

appropriate, thus providing a holistic treatment approach. The most common female sexual difficulties are sexual/genital pain, sexual interest/arousal disorder and non-orgasmic response (Basson 2000). The American Diagnostic and Statistical Manual of Mental Disorders (DSM) is the most frequently used and widely adopted diagnostic criteria for sexual difficulties (American Psychiatric Association 2013). The vast majority of knowledge about sexual difficulties has been gathered from research and clinical practice with heterosexual couples. However, the concepts and methods discussed below are highly applicable to those in same sex relationships, but it is important to address any factors unique to a persons' sexual orientation (Nicols 2014).

A predominantly cognitive/behavioural sex therapy programme comprises of: (Hawton 1993).

- Assessment/History (including treatment goal).
- Education.
- Formulation.
- Treatment.

12.1.1.1 Assessment/History

The main focus of assessment/history taking is to identify whether a sexual difficulty is primary or secondary, generalised or situational. It focuses on highlighting the relevant *predisposing, precipitating* ('triggering events') and *maintaining factors. Predisposing* factors relate any negative experiences during childhood or teenage years that could make a person vulnerable to developing a sexual difficulty in later life. *Precipitating* factors or 'triggering events' are related to what was happening at the time sexual problems became apparent, e.g. childbirth, incontinence, menopause, traumatic experiences, work-related stress, relationship distress, bereavement, divorce, commencing medication, surgery or illness. It is important to ask patients about the quality of their sexual relationship before the event, what they first noticed, how the sexual problem developed and the context in which it is experienced. Identifying current *maintaining* factors helps to explain why problems persist long after the original *predisposing* or *precipitating* event.

A common *maintaining* factor for women with sexual difficulties is avoidance of sexual intimacy and affection, which if identified, can be addressed during treatment. Asking specific and detailed questions can highlight *maintaining* factors relatively easily and can be employed in a variety of clinical settings. It should be noted however, that in some complex cases therapy or counselling may need to focus on the *predisposing* or *precipitating* events, if emotional issues related to these are still current and would interfere with a woman's ability to engage in a sex therapy programme. A common example would be post-traumatic stress related to childhood trauma, sexual abuse, sexual assault or bereavement.

Relationship

Questions should focus on current levels of intimate/sexual activity. This identifies issues of avoidance and helps clarify the appropriateness of suggestions given to a couple in the form of homework assignments. Those who have experienced long periods of avoidance generally require more input to re-establish a satisfying sexual relationship. As Masters and Johnson stated, *'there is no such thing as an uninvolved partner in a relationship where sexual dysfunction exists'* (Masters and Johnson 1970). With some couples the starting point of treatment is about creating quality couple time outside of the bedroom. Exploration of a couple's general relationship can establish whether there is significant relational distress or contextual factors such as work-related stress, disability, financial worries, shift work or caring for family members that are significant in *maintaining* sexual difficulties. These could impede therapy and highlight whether a couple need to access relationship counselling in the first instance. Across the UK Relate offers couple and relationship counselling which can be accessed via www.relateorg.uk.

Negative Behaviours

Negative behaviours can arise as a consequence of sexual difficulties. Common behaviours include apologising during sexual activity, arguments and avoidance of any intimate or sexual activity. In general, negative behaviours lead to further failure and dissatisfaction and increase fear and anxiety. Negative behaviours will often contribute to the *maintenance* of sexual difficulties and explaining their role provides the rationale for behaviour change.

Previous Treatments

Questions about any previous treatments psychological or pharmacological, what benefit they had, if any is important. For example, some women treated for post-menopausal vaginal atrophy with local hormonal or non-hormonal vaginal treatment may report a lack of benefit as they continue to experience pain and discomfort despite any evidence of further pathology. In such cases it is essential that questions regarding her general levels of sexual interest/arousal are asked, anxiety about penetration with its negative impact on sexual response is assessed, and pelvic floor muscle dysfunction is considered as each could potentially cause continued vaginal discomfort (Van der Velde and Everaerd 2001). Women who have previously been prescribed vaginal trainers (dilators) with little success need a detailed assessment of how these were used and what guidance, instruction or support was provided as too often in clinical practice these are insufficient to achieve a successful outcome.

12.1.1.2 Medical History

Sexual dysfunction is often multi-factorial, therefore it is necessary to identify all *maintaining* factors including biological factors and prescribed medications. Whilst therapy itself cannot alter physical changes as a result of medication, cancer treatment, diabetes or menopause, etc., it can address the psychological or behavioural consequences.

Goal Setting

Discussing the goal of treatment allows the therapist to ensure that the outcome a woman expects or is hoping for is realistic and achievable. For those with an organic aetiology or sexual difficulties related to physical changes or as the result of medication, the clinician/therapist must ensure that they don't give false reassurance about the outcome of treatment whilst at the same time instilling confidence that improvement is possible by addressing those maintaining factors that are amenable for change. This stage also identifies what treatment interventions are necessary and the level of time and motivation required from the individual or couple.

12.1.1.3 Education

Education is an essential aspect of sex therapy as it helps patients understand how the body works, human sexual response, normalises some of their experiences, especially around age/disease related changes and highlights possible reasons for unsuccessful pharmacological treatment. For women experiencing genital/sexual pain where underlying pathology has been excluded or treated, discussing the role of the pelvic floor is essential. Education provides an opportunity to explain the role of fear and anxiety, a common feature with both organic and psychogenic sexual pain and discomfort particularly related to its impact on arousal and pelvic floor hypertonicity. Performance anxiety is the fear of future pain or failure based on previous experiences and it interferes with sexual arousal, distracts from sensual feelings, undermines sexual self-confidence and ultimately contributes to sexual avoidance (Zilbergeld 1999).

12.1.1.4 Formulation

This has four main purposes:

1. It provides the rationale for the treatment approach.
2. It should provide the couple or individual with further understanding of their difficulties.
3. It can encourage a sense of optimism about the outcome of treatment.
4. It enables the therapist to check that the information obtained during the assessment has been correctly understood.

12.1.1.5 Structured Behavioural Assignments Often Used in Sex Therapy

Sensate Focus

This is perhaps the most widely known behavioural treatment approach for sexual disorders/dysfunction. The rationale is that behaviours which elicit positive emotions, feelings and responses are likely to be continued and repeated, whilst behaviours that evoke negative emotions, feelings and responses are likely to be avoided (Kirana 2013a). It provides:

1. A structured approach that allows a couple to rebuild their intimate and sexual relationship.
2. Follow-up sessions allow for feedback and can be used diagnostically to help tailor further individual or couple assignments.

Depending on the outcome of the assessment process and identification of *maintaining* factors, couples are given specific relaxing/sensual and/or erotic/sexual suggestions to be carried out at home on a regular basis. They are usually asked to abstain from sexual intercourse as this reduces the inhibitory role of anxiety or fear. Ideally therapy should be flexible and creative, giving couple's choice over what they want to do or feel comfortable with. With established couples, finding out what they did together before the onset of the sexual problem is a good way of ensuring that homework suggestions are appropriate for them. If individuals are in a relationship but their partner cannot attend with them, they should be asked to discuss the expectations and rationale of this approach. For women who have experienced sexual/genital pain, especially those in relatively new relationships or who don't feel a very structured approach would be helpful then penetration could be taken off the agenda but any other pleasurable activities encouraged. Being explicit with a partner ensures that boundaries are clear which promotes increased relaxation and arousal. Partners often worry about causing pain which negatively impacts on their own arousal so this enables them to also enjoy a better intimate/sexual experience. Success of this treatment approach requires patient motivation, a good quality relationship where both partners desire a satisfying sexual life (Althof 2010). Women/couples with complex maintaining factors or health issues may require more in-depth psychotherapeutic/medical interventions.

Systematic Desensitisation
Specific individual techniques to address particular problems, such as systemic desensitisation are usually applied in cases where a phobic response to a sexual stimulus is evident. It has been used in the treatment of genital/sexual pain as well as those suffering from generalised fears of penetration (Kirana 2013a). It may include listing a hierarchy of distress responses, various types of exposure to sexual situations, relaxation and anxiety management techniques, mirror work, use of vaginal trainers (dilators), fingers or vibrator. There are very few studies regarding the use of vaginal trainers (dilators) even though they are a well-established treatment option (Hawton 1993; Smith and Gillmer 1998; Goldstein 2000). A survey carried out in 2004 of 211 COSRT (College of Sexual and Relationship Therapy, formally known as BASRT) members concluded that they achieved a success rate of 83.2% when using vaginal trainers as part of a treatment programme for women with vaginismus.

12.1.1.6   Assessment of Sexual Pain
Identify relevant predisposing, precipitating and maintaining factors (including relevant medical factors) and whether the problem is primary or secondary, generalised or situational.

In DSM 5 sexual pain is classified as genito-pelvic pain/penetration disorder (American Psychiatric Association 2013). Pain is often multi-factorial and can be caused by vaginitis, Bartholin gland abscess, episiotomy scarring, sexually transmitted infections, pelvic inflammatory disease, endometriosis, prolapse or vaginal dryness. The most frequent cause in post-menopausal women is vaginal dryness/

atrophy which can be treated with local oestrogen preparations (Lev-Sagie and Nyirjesy 2009). For women not suitable for local oestrogen treatment, a non-hormonal vaginal moisturiser should be suggested. These products help re-hydrate the vagina and can be used alongside a lubricant. Silicone/oil based lubricants make penetration more comfortable and less likely to dry up than water-based products. Sexual/genital pain can also be caused by inhibition due to body image concerns such as incontinence, reduced sexual interest/arousal, infrequent sexual intercourse and pelvic floor hypertonicity. It is essential that all women are given the opportunity to be examined to determine or exclude any underlying pathology and ideally assessed by a specialist physiotherapist. Pelvic floor muscle hypertonus has been demonstrated to contribute to interstitial cystitis (Peters et al. 2007), provoked vulvodynia (Reissing et al. 2005) and generalised vulvodynia (Glazer et al. 1998). Studies have also demonstrated that pelvic floor muscle hyperactivity is a part of an overall response to heightened anxiety (Fitzgerald and Kotarinos 2003). Genital pain may also trigger pelvic floor dyssynergia (Van der Velde and Everaerd 2001). However, the clinical reality is that some women struggle with being examined and in clinical practice the treatment goal for some women is to achieve a genital examination or cervical cytology. The Lamont classification scale (Fig. 12.1) illustrates the wide range of women's responses and can be a useful tool in helping women understand that their fear responses are triggered instinctively and outside of their conscious control and that simply being told to relax will not be sufficient or helpful. The importance of classifying the severity of a woman's response (Fig. 12.1) impacts on the clinician's ability to diagnose and treat vaginismus, and understand her experience (Rosenbaum 2009).

When opening a discussion, it is important that the clinician is relaxed and comfortable talking about sexual issues. A solid understanding of sexual anatomy and sexual response will enable them to be confident and informative, thus ensuring that

---

The Lamont Scale

- **First degree vaginismus** as spasm of the pelvic floor that could be relieved with reassurance and the patient could relax for her examination.

- **Second degree vaginismus,** generalized spasm of the pelvic floor as a steady state despite reassurance, and the patient was unable to relax for the exam.

- **Third degree vaginismus,** the pelvic floor spasm was sufficiently severe that the patient would elevate her buttocks in an attempt to avoid being examined

- **Fourth degree vaginismus,** the most severe form of vaginismus described by Lamont, the patient would totally retreat by elevating the buttocks, moving away from the pelvic exam, and tightly closing the thighs to prevent any examination.

- **Fifth degree vaginismus,** as a visceral reaction manifested by increased adrenalin output and resulting in any of the following: Increased heart rate, palpitations, hyperventilation, trembling, shaking, nausea or vomiting, crying uncontrollably, a feeling of light headedness and fainting, a desire to jump off the table, run away or even attack the doctor[19].

Fig. 12.1 Lamont J. Vaginismus. American Journal of Obstetrics and Gynaecology 1978 131:633–666. (Pacik et al. 2019)

patients find it easy to talk about their sexual concerns. The effectiveness of any intervention depends on the patient having a positive opinion of the clinician.

12.1.1.7 Questions to Consider

'Could you describe the sexual difficulties you're having?' 'It would be really helpful for me to ask you some personal questions so that I can fully understand the difficulties you have'

- Do they have periods? If so do, can they use tampons?
- If no, have they ever tried to using them? What happened?
- Have they ever had a cervical cytology or been examined? If yes, what happened?
- Do they attempt penetration (penis, vibrator, finger)?
- Has penetration ever been pain-free? When was the last time?
- If they have penetration, how often and how long does it last?
- If they don't have penetration are they still sexually intimate in other ways?
- When and where do they experience pain?
  (before, on, during or after penetration).
- How would they describe the sensations they feel?
  (sharp, burning, stinging, painful, uncomfortable).
- Does anything make it better or worse?
- Do they feel dry or well lubricated?
- Can they keep their legs open?
- How does their partner respond/react?
- Does their partner experience any sexual difficulties?
- How would they describe their experience of sexual interest/arousal/orgasm?

A basic behavioural treatment strategy for sexual/genital pain which addresses common maintaining factors includes the following:

1. When treating sexual/genital pain it is important to acknowledge sexual comorbidity (Petersen 2013). Using Basson's sexual response model provide education and information about genital/sexual pain, how it impacts negatively on sexual interest/arousal/orgasm or how changes in sexual interest/arousal can trigger discomfort during penetration which if unaddressed and persistent can result in pelvic floor dysfunction irrespective of the original aetiology.
2. A diagram/model illustrating the pelvic floor muscles is shown alongside a discussion of pelvic floor responses especially during attempted penetration or tampon use. This is invaluable in helping women make sense of their pain experience and provides rationale for using vaginal trainers (dilators) as part of the treatment process.
3. Instruction on breathing exercises and pelvic floor release/relax techniques are taught—which has not been validated but used extensively in clinical practice with positive results.

4. Information on resources—www.vaginismus.com, 'The wonder down under' by Nina 'Womanhood: The Bare Reality' by Laura Dodsworth.
5. Exposure/desensitisation exercises using finger, vibrator, vaginal trainer (dilator) or tampons (instructions are provided on the handout mentioned above).
6. Discuss penetration positions, for those that are unsure which would be most comfortable or if they feel shy or unsure suggest they practise or rehearse different positions with their clothes on initially this can help them discover what is practical and comfortable.
7. Cognitive restructuring (i.e. replacing unrealistic/irrational beliefs about pain, penetration and sexual functioning), for example when using the vaginal trainers it is 'normal' to feel a stretching sensation or challenging beliefs about sexual interest/arousal using Basson's model of female sexual response.
8. Relaxation/meditation/distraction techniques—to manage anxiety generally or to use prior/with/during or after any form of penetration or sexual intimacy. YouTube has an enormous selection available and Mindfulness Apps like 'Smiling Mind', 'Headspace' or 'Calm' are often suggested.
9. Getting 'your mind on your side'—rehearsing coping self-statements that challenge negative thoughts with positive statements such as 'now I know that it's my pelvic floor muscles that are causing my pain I can consciously learn to control and relax them'.
10. Communication skills specifically related to romantic/sexual partners. If a woman is in a relationship, then there needs to be a discussion regarding their current sexual/intimate activity, such clear boundaries about what activity should be encouraged or included as it is difficult to experience good levels of sexual arousal when we are anxious or afraid so suggestions that increase arousal and psychosexual skills are very important.
11. At the end of their first clinical session most women are given the smallest vaginal trainer (dilator) along with a silicone-based lubricant. If a woman is reluctant to use a vaginal trainer (dilator), they could consider using a cotton bud, their own or their partner's finger or in some cases a small vibrator. The starting point for those with strong fear/panic responses (refer Lamont scale) who struggle to keep their legs open can be given adductor stretching exercises (Amy 2009). Sometimes we suggest mirror work to familiarise herself with her genital area or with her legs open place her hand regularly in-between her legs over underwear to begin with and then under.

Follow-up appointments are used to take feedback on the success or failure of a woman's ability to engage with the treatment plan and adjustments made where necessary, further steps discussed and the next size trainer given (if appropriate). Whilst a woman's ability to increase size is important, frequency of use is crucial as this reduces anxiety thereby helping to reduce/retrain the muscular responses. At some point a discussion will take place regarding the benefits of using a small sized vibrator to help with both physiological arousal and muscular relaxation when used in a circular motion at the introitus. For women who experience reduced sensation related to medical treatment or menopausal changes, it can be helpful to use a vibrator or clitoral suction device for a couple of minutes daily to improve the vascular response and provide nerve stimulation and whilst there is no guarantee of full restoration of sensation, this can facilitate some improvement.

Using the vaginal trainers (dilators) in this way can be sufficient for some women to achieve penetration but for others specific couple suggestions may be needed such as using the trainer or vibrator together, thus allowing a women to accommodate feelings of less control. Other techniques such as outercourse, where a partner simulates the movement of penetration in-between a woman's legs, vaginal containment whereby a penis or vibrator is inserted vaginally with no movement initially and then minimal movement initiated by the woman, thus helping to build couple confidence in a structured way (Hawton 1993). Some women also prefer to use a buffer initially that prevents deep penetration and there are a range of products on the market, e.g. Ohnut. Also available are a wide variety of vaginal trainers (dilators) to choose from, the main differences are related to the number of different sizes in a set and the material they are made from, certainly silicone trainers are softer than hard plastic ones but the benefit of Amielle Comfort in clinical practice is that a box of one size can be purchased and given individually, thus preventing fear and anxiety related to the larger sizes. This product has 5 different sizes but before giving the largest size, enquire about a partner's erect size, if he is similar in size then this stage may not be necessary. In our clinical experience we have found that some patients do not always fit neatly into this treatment programme and it is necessary to develop a flexible attitude and tailor the treatment to the needs of each patient, whilst making pain and their sexual function the central focus of therapy.

12.1.1.8 Assessment of Sexual Interest/Arousal
Identify relevant predisposing, precipitating and maintaining factors (including medical factors) and enquire whether the problem is primary or secondary, generalised or situational.

The DSM-5 term for female sexual desire problems is sexual interest/arousal disorder (American Psychiatric Association 2013). Desire may be physically impaired through hormonal changes, side effects of medications, illness or surgery. Psychological factors such as stress, internal conflicts, anger, depression, low self-esteem, anxiety and persistent symptoms from prior traumatic experiences can inhibit sexual interest/arousal. Sexual ignorance religious prohibition, hostility between partners, destructive behaviour patterns and fatigue are also factors associated with this disorder. Loss of sexual interest/arousal and an inability to orgasm can be secondary to problems with sexual/genital pain or an inability to become orgasmic. The standard narrative of sexual interest or desire is that it is spontaneous and just appears but some women only feel interest or want sex after intimate/sexy or arousing touch is already happening. They are normal, which means a lack of spontaneous desire is not, in itself dysfunctional. These women have 'responsive desire' rather than 'spontaneous desire'; they just need more than the sight of someone attractive to feel sexual interest or become aroused. For others sexual desire is context dependant so if their partner approaches them at night when they feel tired or stressed the outcome may be a negative one but the same approach in the morning after a good night's sleep might be very different. Women can feel relieved when they realise that responsive or context sensitive desire is normal and that they just need more of a reason to be sexual than those with 'spontaneous desire'.

12.1.1.9 Questions to Consider

'Can you describe the sexual difficulties you are having'? 'In order for me to help you, I need to ask you some personal questions, is that okay?'

- How long have they had a problem?
- If there are medical issues how would they describe their sexual/intimate relationship prior to this?
- When was the last time they were sexual with her partner? And before that?
- Ask about distracting thoughts prior to or during sexual intimacy.
- Ask about sexual skills, sexual stimuli and context, including interaction in the preceding hours.
- Do they masturbate?
- Have they tried any previous treatments? (Check compliance/benefit).
- Assess 'why now' and motivation for treatment.
- How would they describe their general relationship?
- Do they have fun together?
- What about emotional intimacy?
- How has each partner responded to the problem?
- Does their partner experience any sexual difficulties.

A basic behavioural treatment strategy for absent or reduced sexual interest/arousal or an inability to orgasm includes the following:

1. Using Basson's sexual response model to provide education and information about female sexual response and the concept of 'responsive desire'. If there are any relevant medical/biological factors that could impact on a women's sexual response, these need to be discussed, including the impact of various chronic diseases. The mechanisms involved can be separated into biological causes that interfere directly with the physiology of the central and peripheral sexual response, and the psychological consequences of being ill (Kirana 2013b).
2. Education regarding female orgasm—An orgasm occurs after sufficient sexual arousal and stimulation of the clitoris is required for the majority of women. Only 30% of women are reliably orgasmic from vaginal penetration alone whilst the remaining 70% are sometimes, rarely or never orgasmic in this way (Nagoski 2017). The physical impact of childbirth, prolapse and menopause can impact negatively on a woman's ability to enjoy orgasmic responses with penetration alone. Information is provided on sex toys, vibrators and clitoral suction devices and how these can be used to enhance pleasure.
3. Identify accelerators and brakes

In her book 'Come as you are' Emily Nagoski introduces the concept of 'Sexual Excitation' and 'Sexual Inhibitory Systems'. This helps women identify their own individual accelerators that 'trigger' sexual interest/arousal and relevant sexual brakes that inhibit their sexual responses. The 'Sexual Temperament Questionnaire' she describes helps women distinguish between their accelerators and brakes, what activates them and how sensitive they are.

4. Context Exercise

This exercise illustrates the importance of context which may be relevant for some women.

Think of a past positive sexual encounter/experience and describe it with as many relevant details that you can recall that includes the following:

1. Mental and physical well-being.
2. Partner characteristics.
3. Relationship characteristics.
4. Setting.
5. Other life circumstances.
6. Things you did.

Next repeat the exercise but this time consider a past negative sexual experience, the focus should be on a situation that you didn't really enjoy rather than something bad or traumatic.

5. Discovering Pleasure

Mindfulness exercises for sexual interest/arousal problems teach women to use sustained attentional focus to bring sensory information, both sexual and not into their awareness. For women who experience inhibited orgasm, strategies like 'orgasmic yoga' or therapeutic masturbation can be introduced (Nagoski 2017). Websites such as www.omgyes.com explore the latest science on female sexual pleasure and what women find sexually arousing. Games, sex/intimacy apps introduce new ideas and listening to erotic podcasts can 'trigger' sexual interest and identify accelerators.

6. Information on strengthening and maintaining a healthy pelvic floor (for women with a normal or weak pelvic floor).

7. Couple Communication Exercise. The focus is to encourage couples to talk and listen to each other. Set aside 20 min every day, each partner has 10 min talk about something important to them whilst the other listens. A way to check that what has been said has been understood is for the listener to repeat back what they have heard. The aim is not to offer solutions but to actively listen and accept that is how a partner feels. In the first instance it is often wise to choose less emotive subjects to begin with.

8. Sensate Focus—for those couples who would benefit from a more structured approach (described earlier in this chapter) to rebuild their intimate/sexual relationship.

Fig. 12.2 Annon J. The PLISSIT Model: A proposed scheme for the behavioural treatment of sexual problems. Journal Sex Education & Therapy, 1976 2:1–15

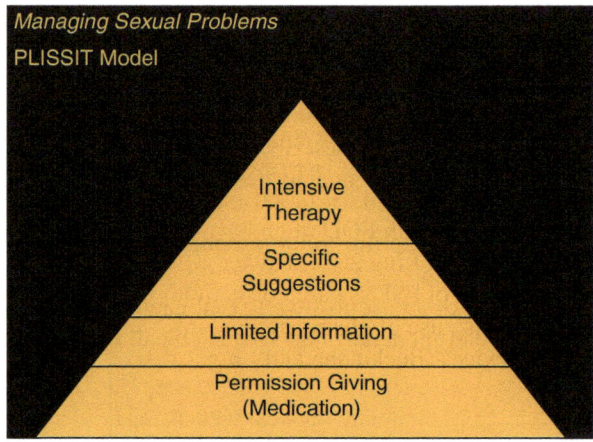

12.1.1.10   PLISSIT: A Sexuality Assessment and Intervention Tool

Annon's PLISSIT model (Fig. 12.2) was developed in the mid-1970s and is still used today; it is a tool for both assessing and managing patients with sexual concerns or difficulties and can be used in a range of clinical specialities. It recognises that the needs of men and women with sexual problems differ due to variable degrees of psychosocial and medical complexity.

PLISSIT is an acronym for the following:
- **P: *Permission.*** Discussing potential sexual changes whilst also addressing disease, cancer or surgical-related changes, gives the patient *permission* to discuss any concerns they have currently or to do so at a later date.
- **LI: *Limited information.*** Give the patient *limited information* about the sexual changes that can stem from their treatment and the basic facts about female sexual response, challenge myths and unrealistic expectations about the norms of sexual functioning and behaviours. Information need not be comprehensive but limited to specific problem areas. On-line help and resources can be recommended such as www.sexualadviceassociation.co.uk and www.menopausedoctor.co.uk
- **SS: *Specific suggestions.*** Make *specific suggestions* that address sexual dysfunction. Such input is largely based on common sense and may only require a couple of sessions. A follow-up appointment is useful to identify the outcome of any initial input and if necessary referral on for sex therapy or counselling.
- **IT: *Intensive therapy.*** If the patient's needs are complex, then an onward referral may be necessary. Information about sex and relationship therapy and how to access NHS/private therapists can be found on the College of Sexual and Relationship Therapy website at www.cosrt.org.uk. Availability of clinicians trained via the Institute of Psychosexual Medicine can be found at www.ipm.org.uk.

12.2   Conclusion

Psychosexual therapy can assess and treat women who experience problems with genital/sexual pain, sexual interest/arousal difficulties and non-orgasmic response. The cognitive behavioural interventions used address the components of a psycho-biological model of sexual function and there is growing scientific evidence supporting the effectiveness of psychological and pelvic floor rehabilitation for the treatment of genital/sexual pain (Bergeron et al. 2009). For all women a multi-disciplinary team approach is strongly recommended and essential when biological factors are present. Provision of psychosexual therapy is not always available. For those services that do exist, not all have sufficient capacity or knowledge to work with women with complex medical issues, therefore it is essential that issues with sexual function are addressed in all specialities where sexual problems are likely to result from disease, illness or surgery; in such cases Annon's model can be utilised (Fig. 12.2). Intervention at the earliest opportunity can prevent more complex problems from developing. The long-term impact of sexual dysfunction can be devastating for both the individual and their partner and rob them of the most intimate part of their relationship. Therefore helping women maintain or restore their sexual functioning is not a lifestyle issue but a quality of life issue and all health care professionals have a major role in providing an opportunity for early discussion and treatment of sexual difficulties.

References

Althof S (2010) What's new in sex therapy? J Sex Med 7(1):5–13
American Psychiatric Association (2013) Diagnostic and statistical manual of mental disorders, 5th edn. American Psychiatric Press, Washington, DC
Amy S (2009) Heal pelvic pain. McGraw-Hill, New York
Basson R (2000) The female sexual response: a different model. J Sex Marital Ther 26:51–65
Bergeron S, Landy T, Leclerc B (2009) Cognitive-behavioural, physical therapy and alternative treatments for dyspareunia. In: Goldstein A, Pukhall C, Goldstein I (eds) Female sexual pain disorders. Wiley Blackwell, Chichester, pp 150–155
Fitzgerald MP, Kotarinos R (2003) Rehabilitation of the short pelvic floor. Int Urogynaecol J 4:261–268
Glazer HI, Jantos M, Hartmann EH, Swencionis C (1998) Electromyographic comparisons of the pelvic floor in women with dysesthetic vulvodynia and asymptomatic women. J Reprod Med 43(11):959–962
Goldstein I (2000) Int J Impot Res 12:S152–S157
Hawton K (1993) Sex therapy a practical guide. Oxford University Press, Oxford
Kirana E (2013a) Psychosexual treatment methods in sexual medicine. In: Kirana PS, Tripoldi R, Reisman Y, Porst H (eds) The EFS & ESSM sullabus of clinical sexology. Medix, Amsterdam
Kirana E (2013b) Sexual desire disorders in women. In: Reisman Y, Porst H (eds) The ESSM syllabus of sexual medicine. Medix, Amsterdam
Lev-Sagie A, Nyirjesy P (2009) Noninfectious vaginitis. In: Goldstein A, Pukhall C, Goldstein I (eds) Female sexual pain disorders. Wiley Blackwell, Chichester
Masters WH, Johnson VE (1970) Human sexual inadequacy. Churchill, London
Nagoski E (2017) Come as you are. Scribe, London

Nicols M (2014) Therapy with LBGTQ clients. In: Binik Y, Hall K (eds) Principles and practice of sex therapy. Guilford, New York, pp 309–333

Pacik PT, Babb CR, Polio A et al (2019) Case series: redefining severe grade 5 vaginismus. Sex Med 7:489–497

Peters KM et al (2007) Prevalence of pelvic floor dysfunction in patients with interstitial cystitis. Urology 70:16–18

Petersen C (2013) Sexual pain disorders. In: Reisman Y, Porst H (eds) The ESSM syllabus of sexual medicine. Medix, Amsterdam

Reissing ED, Brown C, Lord MJ, Binik YM, Khalife S (2005) Pelvic floor muscle functioning in women with vulvar vestibulitis syndrome. J Psychosom Obstet Gynecol 26(2):107–113

Rosenbaum TY (2009) Physical therapy evaluation of dyspareunia. Female sexual pain disorders: evaluation and management. Wiley-Blackwell, Oxford, pp 27–31

Smith KM, Gillmer MD (1998) Amielle vaginal trainers—a patient evaluation. J Obstet Gynaecol 18(2):146–147

Van der Velde J, Everaerd W (2001) The relationship between involuntary pelvic floor muscle activity, muscle awareness and experienced threat in women with and without vaginismus. Behav Res Ther 39:395

Zilbergeld B (1999) The new male sexuality. Bantam, New York

Physical Therapies

13

Bary Berghmans

13.1 Brief Summary

Physiotherapy can contribute significantly to the multidisciplinary assessment and treatment of women with chronic pelvic pain and sexual dysfunctions.

13.2 Introduction

Chronic pelvic pain (CPP) is defined as abdominal pain below the umbilicus for at least 6 months duration (American Psychiatric Association 2013). It is a complex and confusing health problem affecting the quality of life of many women suffering from several urogynaecological disorders (Engeler et al. 2017), often resulting in depression, anxiety and fatique (Laursen et al. 2005).

CPP, with its basis in the central nervous system, involves emotional, cognitive, behavioural and sexual responses (Hoffman 2011). Chronic pelvic pain syndrome (CPPS) is CPP without a proven infection or obvious local pathology and is related to symptoms suggestive of lower urinary tract, bowel, gynaecological and sexual dysfunctions (Laursen et al. 2005).

The sensation and intensity of pain often do not correspond with the identified lesion location, but are felt elsewhere in the body leading to a wide array of musculoskeletal, myofascial disorders and sexual dysfunctions (Hoffman 2011). So,

Notice
Manuscript related to the 13th Ulf Umsten lecture on the 22nd of June, during the 42th IUGA Annual Meeting, Vancouver, Canada.

B. Berghmans (✉)
Pelvic Care Center Maastricht, Maastricht University Medical Centre,
Maastricht, The Netherlands
e-mail: bary.berghmans@maastrichtuniversity.nl

CPP(S) usually coexists with chronic pelvic floor dysfunction, with in most cases the presence of physical findings (Hartmann and Sarto 2014).

13.3 Pathophysiology

The underlying mechanism for this phenomena is partially explained by the following: repeated or prolonged somatic and visceral sensory input of nociceptors (='pain receptor': a sensory neuron that responds to damaging or potentially damaging stimuli by sending 'possible threat' signals to the spinal cord and the brain) results in lowering of their activation treshold, and sensitization of previously non-involved afferent nerve fibres. This is called peripheral sensitization (Willard 2008). Initially, functionally 'silent' fibres may be activated after being sufficiently sensitized by exciting stimuli, increasing the excitability of nociceptors (Aredo et al. 2017).

The electrical impulses initiate neurotransmitter release from nociceptor central terminals which propogate the signal across synapses to the dorsal horn neurons. Greater stimulus intensities are associated with greater release of neuropeptides, including substance P, from central terminals of C-fibres. This mechanism generates a greater postsynaptic response.

This intense afferent bombardement of noxious information through the viscerosomatic convergence and ongoing somatosensoric input from muscle and skin at the dorsal horn of a segment in the spinal cord leads to central sensitization perceived in the brain as prolonged intense pain (Hoffman 2011).

With central sensitization initiation, amplification and perputuation of pain, perception will become manifest as allodynia (a condition where pain is caused by a stimulus that does not normally elicit pain), hyperalgesia and referred pain.

The convergence of neural inputs often hinders precise localization and discrimination of sensory information. It also forms the basis for referred pain, and explains why visceral pathologies are commonly felt as pain in somatic structures, innervated by the same spinal segment (the pelvic floor muscles in particular). Furthermore, since visceral afferent fibres terminate over several spinal segments above and below the segment level of input, referred pain may be present in areas remote from the affected visceral organ.

This upregulation of the sensory system further effects interneurons which connect to alpha and gamma motoneurons leading to segmental overactivity of pelvic floor muscles, spasm and contracture. This pelvic floor dysfunction and myofascial pain can then lead to sexual dysfunction such as dyspareunia or vaginismus as the pelvic floor muscles tighten becoming inflexible and incapacable of accomodating the partner's penis during intercourse.

Myofascial pain is an expression of the dysfunction in the muscle and surrounding myofascial/connective tissue (Aredo et al. 2017). According to Simons et al. (Simons 1996), myofascial pain has a lifetime prevalence of up to 85% in the general population. Nevertheless, physicians have underdiagnosed and often overlooked this health problem. The presence of myofascial triggerpoints (MTrPs) in the symptomatic region is a distinctive feature. MTrPs are small, palpable, hyperirritable nodules located on taut bands of skeletal muscle in an area of sustained contracture (Simons et al. 1999).

MTrPs can be active or latent. Active refers to spontaneously painful areas that do not require physical stimuli, whereas latent are painful only upon physical palpation. Their patterns of referred pain are often predictable and can be documented by anatomical mapping. MTrPs may also cause motor and autonomic disturbances, they can affect the function of visceral organs (Simons et al. 1999). MTrPs are commonly found in many chronic pain conditions, and, when active, typically present as a regional pain syndrome (Aredo et al. 2017).

Simons et al. (1992) noted that in the pelvis minor MTrPs can be found in the vagina, anorectum, urethra, pubic bone, vagina, coccyx, abdomen, lower back and backside of thighs. MTrPs may also refer pain from these muscles back to the pelvic region making myofascial pelvic pain difficult to localize (Pastore and Katzman 2012). Women suffering from myofascial pelvic pain often demonstrate symptoms of dyspareunia, painful urination (dysuria) and difficulty in defecating (dyschezia) though these symptoms may be expressions of other, non-related, pelvic floor or pelvic viscera problems (Simons et al. 1992).

Pelvic floor related sexual dysfunctions are vaginismus, dyspareunia and (chronic) pelvic pain. Many authors report that in patients with CPP and/or sexual dysfunction the role of the pelvic floor is of the utmost importance (Knoepp et al. 2010; Faubion et al. 2012; Fashokun et al. 2013). In 57% of women, with an overactive pelvic floor, dyspareunia has been reported and is felt to be secondary to stretching of shortened pelvic floor muscles, stimulation of painful regions and/or local adhesions, fibrosis or organ dysfunctions (Kotarinos 2003). Because pelvic pain following sexual activity is often sustained for up to 3 days (Salonia et al. 2004), these symptoms can have a large negative impact on the integrity of physical relationships and a women's quality of life inducing feelings of fear, anxiety and depression (Lahaie et al. 2015).

Considering that there is a clear and deep relationship between pelvic floor muscle disorders, (C)PP(S) and female sexual dysfunctions, one would expect an important role for physiotherapy in these patients but in fact the opposite is true. In relevant clinical practice, physiotherapy still seems to be a widely underused strategy, an untapped resource, to decrease CPP and to regain sexual function.

13.4   Hypothesis

In this chapter we hypothesize that in current daily clinical practice physiotherapy should have a place in the multidisciplinary approach to women with CPP(S) and sexual dysfunction.

13.5   Methods

To support our hypothesis relevant literature analysed carrying out a computer-aided and manual search and methodological quality assessment for meta-analyses, systematic reviews and RCTs published between 1990 and 2019 related to physiotherapeutic assessment and treatment of pelvic pain and/or female sexual dysfunctions. Existing classification and models of assessment and interventions used by other relevant healthcare professionals were reviewed. Keywords defined were '(chronic) pelvic pain', 'sexual dysfunction', 'vulvodynia', 'vestibulodynia', 'dyspareunia', 'vaginism', 'sensitization', 'physiotherapy' and 'multidisciplinary'. Besides this, key-opinion leaders from gynaecology, urology, sexology and physiotherapy, all well-known experts in the field, were interviewed about their opinion and clinical expertise.

13.6 Results

The literature search revealed 118 studies. 37 met our criteria, of which there were no meta-analyses, 28 (systematic) reviews, and 9 RCTs.

13.6.1 Classifications and Models

In order to more reliably diagnose female sexual dysfunction, the American Physiatric Association's (APA) Diagnostic and Statistical Manual of Mental Disorders 5® (DSM-V) classifies *mental* disorders with associated criteria (American Psychiatric Association 2013). These classifications include psychogenic and organic causes of abnormal desire, arousal, orgasm and sexual pain disorders. This diagnostic and classification system is based on physiologic as well as psychologic pathophysiology, and includes a personal distress criterion for most diagnoses. Although the APA recognizes that female sexual dysfunction for many women is *physically* disconcerting (American Psychiatric Association 2013), the DSM classifications are specifically limited to psychiatric disorders and are not intended to be used for evaluating or differentiating the physical aspects of sexual dysfunction (American Psychiatric Association 2013). Moreover, sexual disorders, such as dyspareunia and vaginism, are typically diagnosed independent of aetiology, which may be largely or entirely physical in some instances.

Dyspareunia and vaginismus both are part of the spectrum of painful intercourse, the difference being a matter of severity (Crowley et al. 2009). The DSM-V classification stresses that dyspareunia and vaginismus are penetration disorders in that any form of vaginal penetration such as with tampons, finger, vaginal dilators, gynaecological examinations, and intercourse are painful (dyspareunia and vaginismus) or impossible (vaginismus). These conditions are still often underdiagnosed and therefore inadequately treated, despite affecting millions of women worldwide (Pacik 2014). Moreover, psychiatrists and psychologists find it difficult to differentiate between dyspareunia and vaginismus (American Psychiatric Association 2013). The prevalence of dyspareunia and vaginismus is about 8–16%, mostly involving the diagnoses of vulvar vestibulitis or vulvodynia (Engman et al. 2004). Other literature estimates the prevalence of female sexual dysfunction resulting from chronic pelvic and sexual pain to be 26% (range 7 to 58%) (Hayes et al. 2006). Provoked vestibulodynia (PVD) is another common subtype of vulvodynia, affecting approximately 12% of women (Harlow and Stewart 2003).

In younger women, vaginismus has been reported to affect up to 21% of women <30 years of age (Laumann et al. 1999), with an cumulative incidence of 10% of women unable to have sexual intercourse because of pain.

So far, gynaecologists and related medical professionals frequently only focused on the assessment, evaluation and treatment of *peripheral* manifestations and location of CPP(S). Central sensitization and myofascial dysfunction are in many cases overlooked probably because of lack of training in the assessment of myofascial dysfunction (Aredo et al. 2017).

Little more than one decade ago physiotherapy for pelvic pain and female sexual dysfunction was almost nonexsistent with only a few studies reporting on this subject. The well-known psychiatrist Rosemary Basson et al. (Basson 2005) categorized the diagnosis and definition of major categories of women's sexual dysfunction and their management. Vaginismus was defined as persisting or recurrent difficulties in allowing vaginal entry of any object, despite the woman's expressed wish to do so. The behavioural component was mentioned as the main source for management without any reference to physiotherapy. For dyspareunia the authors suggested treatment with cyclic antidepressants, with or without pelvic muscle physiotherapy, without any further specification (Basson 2005). Important work by this group introduced the concept of a circular response cycle in women, the 'Female sexual response cycle' (Basson 2001).

They stated that, next to sufficient sexual stimuli and motivation, the women's state of mind, thought processes, beliefs and emotions might be the most important part of the sexual response cycle. The woman most likely would become more aroused and would desire sex more when they were in a safe and secure surrounding and circumstances. They did mention that anxiety or distraction because of pain or discomfort may limit the woman to be open to or agree to have sex, which could hinder sexual arousal and desire. Therefore, in this cycle there are not only psychological factors, but also physiological and physical factors that can play an important role. So, why did they relegate physiotherapy to a minor role in this cycle?

There is a new evolving model in which each individual can be seen as a social-psychosomatic entity with an intricate and variable interaction of physical factors (genetic, phenotypically, biochemical, etc.), psychological factors (mood, personality, behaviour, etc.), and social factors (cultural, familial, socioeconomic, medical, etc.) (Santrock 2007). This recent biopsychosocial model applies to disciplines ranging from medicine to psychology to sociology; its novelty, acceptance and prevalence vary across disciplines and across cultures (Santrock 2007; Penney 2010). However, this model is very useful for the understanding and evaluation of the complexity of pelvic pain and female sexual dysfunctions, which are often multifactorial, requiring a multidisciplinary assessment and approach to treatment.

So far, there has been a tendency to experience pelvic pain, dyspareunia and vaginism as *psychological distress* resulting in the form of somatic or physical symptoms and to give medication or surgical help for these symptoms. The medical doctor, psychiatrist, or psychologist often consider these symptoms to be initiated and/or perpetuated by emotional responses such as anxiety and depression.

Keeping this in mind, in order to answer the question of where physiotherapy should fit in the sex response cycle, first of all, it is important to understand the rationale of and the relationship between the medical ICD-10 and the APA classification DSM-V and the physiotherapists International Classification of Functions (ICF) for (pelvic) physiotherapy (WHO 2018).

Where medical doctors use the ICD-10 to code the diagnoses of pelvic pain and sexual dysfunctions and psychiatrists, psychologists and sexologists use the DSM-V to classify and define pelvic pain and sexual dysfunctions, physiotherapists use the International Classification of Functions (ICF) (Table 13.1) (WHO 2018).

Using the ICF, the physiotherapist tries to influence the *consequences* of pelvic pain and sexual dysfunction on 3 different levels: organ level (impairment/disorder level, e.g. intra-vaginal pain at penetration), personal level (disability level, e.g. inability to have intercourse) and social-societal level (restriction of participation, e.g. avoidance of sexual relationship = behavioural consequence).

Where the DSM-V acts mainly on the psychological aspects of the personal and the social-societal level, with the focus on (the change of inadequate) behaviour, the ICF also incorporates the organ level, local physical disorders or impairments (WHO 2018).

In Basson's sex response cycle (Fig. 13.1), elements such as 'psychological and biological processing', 'arousal and responsive sexual desire', 'multiple reasons and incentives for instigating or agreeing to sex', and 'motivation', require both adequate psychological and physical responses. Local pain or MTrP, overactive pelvic floor muscles, central sensitization related hyperalgesia and anxiety may hinder the mind setting for sex and/or sexual activity. Here, not only psychological counselling and intervention but also (pelvic) physiotherapy may be an important (co-) intervention.

As an example of this interplay, the cause of pelvic pain and dyspareunia might be due to an injury to the pelvic floor muscles, connective tissue or fascia as a result of a (birth) trauma, sexual or physical abuse, or an episiotomy during the vaginal delivery. This can lead to shortened and weak pelvic floor muscle with MTrPs and restriction of connective tissue resulting in chronic pelvic pain and dyspareunia. Ongoing and unresolved local injuries may lead to spinal cord central sensitization and because of dorsal root reflexes at the spinal cord level lead to the development of referred symptoms of frequency, urgency and nocturia and eventual development

Table 13.1 Definitions of the International Classification of Functioning Terms: impairment, disability and restriction in participation

Impairment: Loss or abnormality of psychological, physiological, or anatomical structure or function at organ level
Disability: Restriction or loss of ability of a person to perform functions/activities in a normal manner
Restriction in participation: Disadvantage due to impairment or disability that limits or prevents fulfilment of a normal role (depends on age, sex, sociocultural factors) for the person

Source: WHO-Publication, International Classification of Functioning, Disability and Health (ICF), World Health Organization, Geneva, Switzerland, 2018

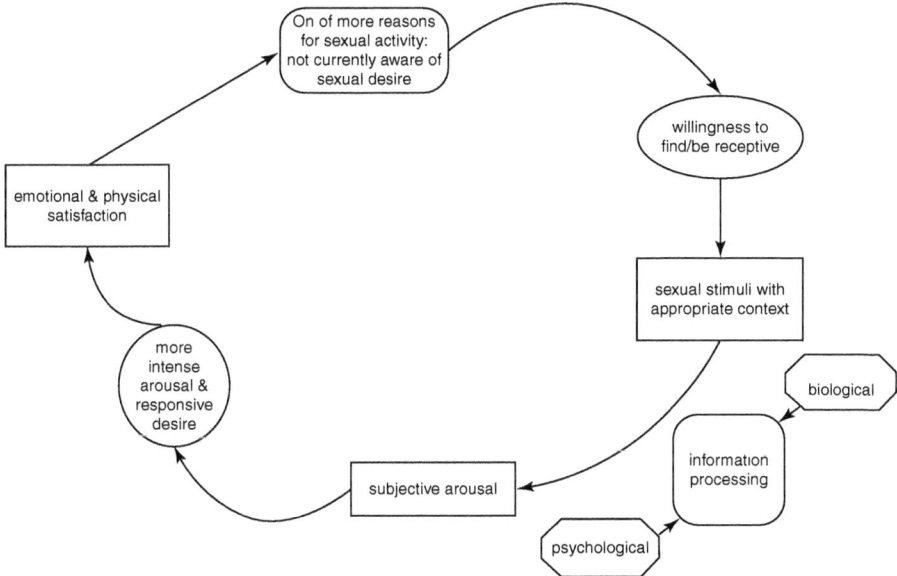

Fig. 13.1 The Female Sexual Response Cycle (adapted from Basson (2001))

of non-infectious cystitis. This, in turn, provokes more pain, urgency, frequency and nocturia, resulting in further contraction/tension of the pelvic floor muscles, with further shortening and restriction of connective tissue (Faubion et al. 2012; Fashokun et al. 2013).

Up to now, it was the rare clinician who, when assessing cystitis, would take into consideration that the cause of the cystitis is related to a latent injury of the pelvic floor with consequential central sensitization and dorsal root reflexes. Most likely, the clinician would rather continue the diagnostic process with more invasive techniques or prescription of medication, instead of referring the patient to pelvic physiotherapy which may be a very reasonable alternative/addition.

Women with pelvic pain and sexual dysfunction constitute a group of patients with significant morbidity. They do not just suffer with pain but with difficulty of walking, maintaining life, work ability and social interactions.

As mentioned before, pelvic pain and female sexual dysfunctions are often related to pelvic floor muscle dysfunction, such as overactive or underactive pelvic floor or coordination disorders. Stress as the central factor provokes a vicious cycle with pain leading to muscle tension, pressure or entrapment of nerves, developing reduced circulation, which results in muscle shortening, leading to restricted movement, creation of MTrPs with again pain as a consequence (Rosenbaum 2011).

The cause of stress and/or pain is not a simple or single problem but complex and multiple. By the time women with CPP are diagnosed with pelvic floor muscle dysfunction, they already have undergone many unsuccessful therapeutic trials that often did not provide adequate relief. According to the interviewed key-opinion leaders, for these women, patient's self-empowerment is essential and the physiotherapy role is critical. It is not just the pelvic floor but the global impact of pain on the body. Many patients will not have only pelvic pain but many other musculoskeletal manifestations. So, the role of physiotherapy is to get to the heart of the matter by starting with the basics of getting the patient to stand, sit and walk properly. In doing so the musculoskeletal impact of decreased strain and improved comfort is the first thing a lot of patients start to notice. Following this the physiotherapist can then move on to working specifically on the pelvic floor. Such a multidisciplinary protocol, with a central role for physiotherapy has been developed at the University College Hospital, London, UK, with reported high levels of clinical efficacy and patient satisfaction (personal communication, Dr. Sohier Elneil, 2017). Physiotherapists need to be trained and skilled not only in how to deal with pain avoidance, using cognitive or behavioural models, but also to actively listen and display empathy for the emotional component of their disease (Rosenbaum 2011).

In case of a referral to a pelvic physiotherapist, an accurate medical diagnosis is very important to determine the severity and impact of the complaints of the patient and to estimate the success or failure of pelvic floor physiotherapy. As mentioned before, in a lot of cases the **presumed** medical diagnosis (also called 'indication') lacks accuracy, confronting the physiotherapists with heterogeneity and unclear grade of severity, which might result in a minor degree of success or even failure. The fact that many women with dyspareunia or vaginismus will have high levels of anxiety in response to a physical examination involving an assessment of the external and internal pelvic structures leads to under-diagnosing conditions (Goldstein et al. 2016).

Relevant scientific studies showed that medical doctors did not specify the location of pain in 93%, duration of pain in 44%, pathology in 74%, co-morbidities in 95%, and additional inclusion/exclusion criteria in 65% of cases referred to physiotherapy (Engeler et al. 2017; Williams et al. 2004). In a review of Kavvadias et al., which included 69 articles, the site of pain was specified in only 45% of the studies, and only 20% of medical doctors performed a digital examination of pelvic MTrPs for diagnosis (Kavvadias et al. 2011).

So, up to now, because of lack of sufficient relevant medical information, referral data and test results, focused physiotherapy was difficult to administer adequately.

Recently, there is a tendency to involve physiotherapists more and more in the multidisciplinary assessment and treatment of female sexual dysfunctions and pain management. Multidisciplinary guidelines (Engeler et al. 2017) and protocols (University College Hospital, 2017) have been developed and are available. The Pain Clinic of the University Medical Center Groningen (UMCG), Groningen, The Netherlands, developed the pain medicine management model. Whereas, in the past, in the case of a pain complaint the patient was assessed by only one medical doctor followed immediately by a treatment, nowadays, the assessment is based on the patient's complaint, and a multidisciplinary approach to both evaluation and treatment is central to the new model. Through a multidisciplinary assessment, including a thorough history, physical exam with additional testing/examination as indicated, the team develops a comprehensive diagnosis that includes a presumed pathophysiology of the (dominant) pain mechanism. The UMCG multidisciplinary pain centre team consists of a medical team (urologist, gynaecologist, surgeon), a psychologist and a physiotherapist. They assess predominant nociceptive, neuro-pathic, non-neuropathic, somatic, visceral and referred neuropathy, evaluating the presence of peripheral and central sensitization, and taking into account any pro-voking and perpetuating biopsychosocial factors in women with CPP and/or sexual dysfunction. The assessment takes 1 h of each of the disciplines (medical doctor, psychologist/psychiatrist/sexologist and physiotherapist). Consequently, the patient can be classified and the plan of care can be tailored (Wijma et al. 2016).

In the next paragraphs, based on relevant literature, key-leader opinion and clini-cal experience, physiotherapeutic assessment and treatment are described and sci-entific evidence discussed.

13.6.2 Physiotherapeutic Assessment and Treatment

Cacchioni et al. looked in detail at sexual therapy for women involving 'body work', i.e. work on people's body involving touch (Cacchioni and Wolkowitz 2011). Women seeking advice for sexual problems usually are assessed and treated by involving close scrutiny, measurement and touch of the genital area by healthcare providers, including the medical doctor and the pelvic physiotherapist (Cacchioni and Wolkowitz 2011). Treatment may also involve instructing the woman in genital self-touch. A good tool for the management of CPP and female sexual dysfunction might be the so-called 'ALLOW' algorithm introduced by Sadovsky and Mulhall (2003). ALLOW is a management plan with 5 steps. Only once the current step has been fulfilled satisfactorily for both the woman and the pelvic physiotherapist, the next step can start.

- Step 1: **A**: **ask** the patient whether you can proceed with the procedures, then.
- Step 2: **L**: **legitimize** each part of the body work in such a way that the patient completely feels in control,
- Step 3: **L**: **limitations** meaning that the pelvic physiotherapist at all time, before start and during the body work is aware of his/her own competence, skills and the patient's emotions and feelings and refers if necessary to another professional,
- Step 4: **O**: **open up** for further discussion and evaluation with the patient and, if necessary, other competent colleagues or other disciplines of the multidisci-plinary team,
- Step 5: **W**: **work together** to develop a treatment plan with the patient and other disciplines.

13.6.3 Physical Exam

Before beginning the physical exam, the pelvic physiotherapist informs the patient about the nature of procedure, to 'make the patient feel comfortable' and to 'set clear boundaries' (Cacchioni and Wolkowitz 2011). Also the pelvic physiotherapist explains the difference between the objectives and execution of the physical exam done by their physician and the physiotherapist. The physiotherapist attends to women's immediate complaints of sexual discomfort or displeasure through forms of body work that encourage women to feel in control during both body work procedures and sexual activities. Patients with female sexual dysfunctions described the body work techniques as therapeutic and empowering. Especially, assessment and treatment modalities with visualization and hands-on care techniques that stimulate reconnection to their bodies, rather than a sensation of objective feelings. These strategies are often highly praised by patients because of the careful, slow, gradual approach which encourages women to be active participants in the overall process (Cacchioni and Wolkowitz 2011).

After a general inspection of posture and stability of spine and pelvis, the physical exam begins with inspection of the abdominal wall and observation of patient's breath while the patient is in supine position. Then inspection of the perineal region will take place, observing the skin (colour, temperature), scars, irregularities, moisture, etc. Next, a neuromuscular exam, assessing dermatomes, myotomes, searching for MTrPs, allodynia (skin rolling test, pinch and roll technique), hyperalgesia (Wartenberg pinwheel), nerve entrapment and pain points will be performed. Muscle activity (tone) of low back, hip, leg and abdominal muscles will be examined, using palpation techniques. Pelvic floor muscle activity (tone), spasm and relaxation will be assessed by internal palpation and/or biofeedback (Aredo et al. 2017; Bo et al. 2017; Fuentes-Marquez et al. 2019).

More detailed information about physiotherapist's physical examination techniques and interpretation can be found elsewhere (Berghmans et al. 2020).

13.6.4 Treatment

Information about the underlying health problem and education of the patient are always the starting point of treatment. The educational component of the intervention includes explanations about CPP pathophysiology and female sexual dysfunctions, the involvement of PFM, healthy vulvovaginal and sexual behaviours, factors influencing pain intensity, relaxation techniques, sexual function and recovery of non-painful sexual activities (Morin et al. 2016).

Physiotherapist-assisted stretching of the muscles of the back, lower extremities and abdomen in addition to nerve gliding to facilitate movement in restricted nerves is important (Goldstein et al. 2016). Next to these stretching exercises strengthening techniques that address muscle weakness, allowing for balance and stability are provided.

As mentioned before, central sensitization and a myofascial source may contribute to CPP and associated sexual dysfunctions. To directly address myofascial pain pelvic physiotherapists use strategies for treatment of MTrPs and pain regions especially those which have been clinically tested and enhanced by scientific studies. Myofascial release techniques involve physiotherapy and manual therapy modalities including deep pressure massage, stretching techniques, joint mobilization, foam rollers (FitzGerald et al. 2012) and other triggerpoint inactivation techniques such as vibration, pincet, transversal or flat palpation (FitzGerald et al. 2012; Anderson et al. 2009) and dry needling (Ay et al. 2010).

About 30 min of each session will be dedicated to these manual techniques to increase flexibility, decrease TRP related pain and tension of pelvic floor muscles and increase balance and stability. Besides these techniques, other pain management strategies, including general and specific respiratory and relaxation exercises aim to enhance patient's self-management and self-empowerment (Pastore and Katzman 2012; Desai et al. 2013). Aredo et al. reported that 'this dual approach addresses physiological and psychological components of chronic myofascial pain, alleviates MTrP related pain, and furnishes patients with coping strategies to redirect their focus during a painful episode' (Aredo et al. 2017).

Other frequently used treatment modalities are pain management programmes to promote behaviour change (Jensen et al. 1991), pelvic floor muscle training (Clemens et al. 2000; Berghmans 2017), biofeedback, electrical stimulation (Srinivasan et al. 2007), balloons and vaginal dilitators of vaginal tissues (Gentilcore-Saulnier et al. 2010).

Goldstein et al. (2016) described a programme of pelvic floor muscle training for vulvodynia. Pelvic and core mobilization and stabilization techniques, connective tissue, visceral, and neural mobilization were used as well as internal and external myofascial trigger point release. Biofeedback and electrical stimulation assisted in decreasing tender points and decrease of tissue restrictions. The aim was to restore the proper length of the pelvic floor muscles and tissues, decreasing neural tension, and decreasing dyspareunia. Vaginal dilators can be recommended to normalize the tone of the muscles, desensitize hypersensitive areas of the vulva and vagina, and restore sexual function (Kellogg-Spadt et al. 2012).

The daily home maintenance programme involves relaxation and respiratory exercises, pelvic floor muscles training to control their functions, stretching techniques and the use of vaginal dilatators, if indicated (Morin et al. 2016).

13.7 Scientific Evidence for Pelvic Physiotherapy

Recently, more qualitative studies have been published on the effects of pelvic physiotherapy for CPP and female sexual dysfunctions. Weiss et al. (2012) reported that regular, both in-clinic and at home PFM training augments the support function of the pelvic floor, increases blood flow and stimulates PFM proprioception, contributing to more intense orgasm. A review on chronic pelvic floor dysfunction, (Hartmann and Sarto 2014) concluded that referral to a pelvic physiotherapist should occur routinely as part of the multidisciplinary approach for all women who present with any type of vulvovaginal pain. Research indicates that pelvic physiotherapy is safe and effective, and can dramatically improve symptoms related to CPP and chronic PFD. Pelvic physiotherapy stimulates the self-empowerment of women and supports the recovery of function they may have lost due to the pain and dysfunction. Also Sadownik et al. (2012) (qualitative retrospective study), Brotto et al. (2015)

(longitudinal prospective study), Goldstein et al. (2016) (report of the expert committee of the Fourth International Consultation on Sexual Medicine) and Goldfinger et al. (2016) (randomized clinical trial (RCT)) underline the efficacy of pelvic physiotherapy as part of the multidisciplinary approach for CPP and sexual dysfunctions.

Goldstein et al. (2016) stated that physiotherapist-assisted stretching of all muscles related to the pelvis, abdomen. Low back and upper legs, in addition to nerve gliding to facilitate movement in restricted nerves is a necessary condition to improve pelvic floor and sexual dysfunctions. According to the findings of the assessment, the physiotherapist combined stretching exercises with strength training restoring balance and stability, proper length of the pelvic floor muscles and fascial tissues, decreasing neural tension, and decreasing dyspareunia.

In a Randomized Controled Trial (RCT), Goldfinger et al. (2016) investigated effects on provoked vestibulodynia comparing cognitive-behavioural therapy and multimodal physiotherapy. The physiotherapy protocol included education, PFM exercises, manual techniques, surface electromyographic biofeedback, progressive vaginal penetration exercises through the use of four silicone vaginal dilators of varied diameter, stretching of hip muscles, deep breathing and global body relaxation exercises, and pain management techniques. They concluded that both interventions are effective treatment options for women with provoked vestibulodynia.

Sadownik et al. (2012) stated that behaviour change by physiotherapists, empowering the patient's bodily experience through techniques such as graded exposure is an important aspect to improve self-efficacy and decrease overly negative cognitions.

Vaginal electrical stimulation improved the sexual life of women with a pelvic floor dysfunction who scored low on the Female Sexual Function Index (FSFI) (RCT) (Aydın et al. 2015) while transcutaneous electrical nerve stimulation (TENS) was reported to be feasible and beneficial for treatment-resistant provoked vestibulodynia (Vallinga et al. 2015) (longitudinal prospective study). In a RCT among women with pelvic and sexual pain, Zoorob et al. (2015) concluded that pelvic physiotherapy improves sex life and decreases pain equilavent to levator injections. Comparing the effect of physiotherapy with surgery on sexual function in women with PFD, physiotherapy showed to be an appropriate method with similar outcomes (RCT) (Eftekhar et al. 2014).

A randomized clinical trial was conducted among 97 Iranian postmenopausal women, aged 40 to 60 years (Nazarpour et al. 2018). The participants' baseline sexual functions were assessed using the FSFI questionnaire. They were then randomly designated to two groups: (1) the intervention group, which received specific instructions on PFM exercises and was followed up on a weekly basis; and (2) the control group, which received general information on menopause. After 12 weeks, the sexual functions of the participants were reassessed. The significant results in favour of the experimental group led to the conclusion that pelvic floor muscle exercises have the potential to improve the sexual function of postmenopausal women and are thus suggested to be included in healthcare packages designed for postmenopausal women (Nazarpour et al. 2018).

In a RCT including 114 women with urinary incontinence and sexual dysfunction, Jha et al. (2018) compared pelvic floor muscle training and electrostimulation with pelvic floor muscle training alone. Only 64 of 114 finished the study. Based on the Prolapse and Incontinence Sexual function Questionnaire (PISQ) results were similarly effective in both groups which indicated that physiotherapy is beneficial to improve overall sexual function. However, no specific form of physiotherapy appeared to be beneficial over another (Jha et al. 2018).

Ghaderi et al. (2019) evaluated in a RCT including 64 women, comparing electrotherapy, manual therapy and PFM exercises with no treatment, the effects of these pelvic floor rehabilitation techniques on dyspareunia. Evaluations of PFM strength and endurance, sexual function, and pain were made directly before and after 3 months of treatment and at the 3-month follow-up. Between-group changes showed significant improvement in the experimental group in comparison with control group. According to the results, the authors concluded that pelvic floor rehabilitation is an important part of a multidisciplinary treatment approach to dyspareunia (Schvartzman et al. 2019).

Another recent RCT randomized 42 women with dyspareunia to receive pelvic physiotherapy or lower back and abdominal physical therapy Ghaderi et al. (2019). Patients who received pelvic physiotherapy showed significant improvement in pain ($P \leq 0.001$), overall quality-of-life scores ($P \leq 0.001$) and overall sexual function ($P < 0.018$), compared with patients who did not have pelvic floor training Ghaderi et al. (2019).

13.8 Conclusions

CPP and female sexual dysfunctions are prevalent, multifactorial and quality of life threatening health problems. As part of the multidisciplinary team, and because of its holistic and whole-body approach, pelvic physiotherapy can contribute significantly in the assessment and treatment for women with CPP and sexual dysfunction. Clinical and scientific research indicate its efficacy and safety. More high quality RCTs are warranted on several physiotherapeutic treatment modalities and protocols, and to investigate their long-term effects.

The role for pelvic physiotherapy in patients with CPP and sexual dysfunction from an untapped resource towards an integrated part of the treatment is still evolving but remains very promising for all women with CPP and sexual dysfunctions. Adequate and evidence-based knowledge and clinical practical skills together with an empathic attitude of physiotherapists are both challenge and mainstay of current education and training.

Acknowledgements I would like to express my gratitude to Sohier Elneil, PhD MD gynaecologist, Bert Messelink, MD, urologist and sexologist, Fetske Hogen Esch, pelvic physiotherapist, Maura Seleme, PhD pelvic physiotherapist, Nucelio Lemos, PhD MD gynaecologist for their advices and contribution in the realization of this chapter.
Conflict of Interest Statement: none.

References

American Psychiatric Association (2013) Diagnostic and statistical manual of mental disorders, 5th edn. American Psychiatric Association, Arlington, VA

Anderson RU, Sawyer T, Wise D, Morey A, Nathanson BH (2009) Painful myofascial trigger points and pain sites in men with chronic prostatitis/chronic pelvic pain syndrome. J Urol 182(6):2753–2758

Aredo JV, Heyrana KJ, Karp BI, Shah JP, Stratton P (2017) Relating chronic pelvic pain and endometriosis to signs of sensitization and myofascial pain and dysfunction. Semin Reprod Med 35:88–97

Ay S, Evcik D, Tur BS (2010) Comparison of injection methods in myofascial pain syndrome: a randomized controlled trial. Clin Rheumatol 29(1):19–23

Aydın S, Arıoğlu Aydın C, Batmaz G, Dansuk R (2015) Effect of vaginal electrical stimulation on female sexual functions: a randomized study. J Sex Med 12:463–469

Basson R (2001) Human sex-response cycles. J Sex Marital Ther 27(1):33–43

Basson R (2005) Women's sexual dysfunction: revised and expanded definitions. CMAJ 172:1327–1333

Berghmans B (2017) Pelvic floor muscle training: what is important? A mini-review. Obstet Gynecol Int J 6(4):00214. https://doi.org/10.15406/ogij.2017.06.00214

Berghmans B, Seleme MR, Bernards ATM (2020) Physiotherapy assessment for female urinary incontinence. Int Urogynecol J 31:917. https://doi.org/10.1007/s00192-020-04251-2

Bo K, Frawley HC, Haylen BT, Abramov Y, Almeida FG, Berghmans B, Bortolini M, Dumoulin C, Gomes M, McClurg D, Meijlink J, Shelly E, Trabuco E, Walker C, Wells A (2017) An International Urogynecological Association (IUGA)/International Continence Society (ICS) joint report on the terminology for the conservative and nonpharmacological management of female pelvic floor dysfunction. Int Urogynecol J 28(2):191–213. Epub 2016 Dec 5. https://doi.org/10.1007/s00192-016-3123-4

Brotto LA, Yong P, Smith KB, Sadownik LA (2015) Impact of a multidisciplinary vulvodynia program on sexual functioning and dyspareunia. J Sex Med 12:238–247

Cacchioni T, Wolkowitz C (2011) Treating women's sexual difficulties: the body work of sexual therapy. Sociol Health Illn 33(2):266–279. ISSN 0141–9889. https://doi.org/10.1111/j.1467-9566.2010.01288.x

Clemens JQ, Nadler RB, Schaeffer AJ, Belani J, Albaugh J, Bushman W (2000) Biofeedback, pelvic floor re-education, and bladder training for male chronic pelvic pain syndrome. Urology 56(6):951–955

Crowley T, Goldmeier D, Hiller J (2009) Diagnosing and managing vaginismus. BMJ 338:b2284

Desai MJ, Bean MC, Heckman TW, Jayaseelan D, Moats N, Nava A (2013) Treatment of myofascial pain. Pain Manag 3(1):67–79

Eftekhar T, Sohrabi M, Haghollahi F, Shariat M, Miri E (2014) Comparison effect of physiotherapy with surgery on sexual function in patients with pelvic floor disorder: a randomized clinical trial. Iran J Reprod Med 12(1):7–14

Engeler D, Baranowski AP, Borovicka J, Cottrell AM, Dinis-Oliveira P, Elneil S, Hughes J, Messelink EJ, Williams AC (2017) Guidelines Associates: Goonewardene S, Schneider MP. EAU guidelines on chronic pelvic pain. Limited update March 2017

Engman M, Lindehammar H, Wijma B (2004) Surface electromyography diagnostics in women with partial vaginismus with or without vulvar vestibulitis and in asymptomatic women. J Psychosom Obstet Gynaecol 25(3–4):281–294

Fashokun TB, Harvie HS, Schimpf MO, Olivera CK, Epstein LB, Jean-Michel M, Rooney KE, Balgobin S, Ibeanu OA, Gala RB, Rogers RG, Society of Gynecologic Surgeons' Fellows' Pelvic Research Network (2013) Sexual activity and function in women with and without pelvic floor disorders. Int Urogynecol J 24(1):91–97

Faubion SS, Shuster LT, Bharucha AE (2012) Recognition and management of nonrelaxing pelvic floor dysfunction. Mayo Clin Proc 87(2):187–193

FitzGerald MP, Payne CK, Lukacz ES, Yang CC, Peters KM, Chai TC, Nickel JC, Hanno PM, Kreder KJ, Burks DA, Mayer R, Kotarinos R, Fortman C, Allen TM, Fraser L, Mason-Cover M, Furey C, Odabachian L, Sanfield A, Chu J, Huestis K, Tata GE, Dugan N, Sheth H, Bewyer K, Anaeme A, Newton K, Featherstone W, Halle-Podell R, Cen L, Landis JR, Propert KJ, Foster HE Jr, Kusek JW, Nyberg LM, Interstitial Cystitis Collaborative Research Network (2012) Randomized multicenter clinical trial of myofascial physical therapy in women with interstitial cystitis/painful bladder syndrome and pelvic floor tenderness. J Urol 187(6):2113–2118

Fuentes-Marquez P, Valenza MC, Cabrera-Martos I, Rıos-Sanchez A, Ocon-Hernandez O (2019) Trigger points, pressure pain Hyperalgesia, and Mechanosensitivity of neural tissue in women with chronic pelvic pain. Pain Med 20:5–13

Gentilcore-Saulnier E, McLean L, Goldfinger C et al (2010) Pelvic floor muscle assessment outcomes in women with and without provoked vestibulodynia and the impact of a physical therapy program. J Sex Med 7:1003e22

Ghaderi F, Bastani P, Hajebrahimi S, Jafarabadi MA, Berghmans B. Pelvic floor rehabilitation in the treatment of women with dyspareunia: a randomized controlled clinical trial. Int Urogynecol J. 2019. https://doi.org/10.1007/s00192-019-04019-3. PMID 31286158; PMCID: PMC6834927

Goldfinger C, Pukall CF, Thibault-Gagnon S, McLean L, Chamberlain S (2016) Effectiveness of cognitive-behavioral therapy and physical therapy for provoked vestibulodynia: a randomized pilot study. J Sex Med 13:88–94

Goldstein AT, Pukall CF, Brown C, PharmD BS, Stein A, Kellogg-Spadt S (2016) Vulvodynia: assessment and treatment. J Sex Med 13:572–590

Harlow BL, Stewart EG (2003) A population-based assessment of chronic unexplained vulvar pain: have we underestimated the prevalence of vulvodynia? J Am Med Womens Assoc 58:82

Hartmann D, Sarton J (2014) Chronic pelvic floor dysfunction. Best Practice & Research Clinical Obstetrics and Gynaecology 28:977–990

Hayes RD, Bennett CM, Fairley CK et al (2006) What can prevalence studies tell us about female sexual difficulty and dysfunction? J Sex Med 3(4):589–595

Hoffman D (2011) Understanding multisymptom presentations in chronic pelvic pain: the interrelationships between the viscera and myofascial pelvic floor dysfunction. Pain Headache Rep 15:343–346

Hsu AL, Sinaii N, Segars J, Nieman LK, Stratton P (2011) Relating pelvic pain location to surgical findings of endometriosis. Obstet Gynecol 118(2 Pt 1):223–230

Jensen MP, Turner JA, Romano JM (1991) Self-efficacy and outcome expectancies: relationship to chronic pain coping strategies and adjustment. Pain 44(3):263–269

Jha S, Walters SJ, Bortolami O, Dixon S, Alshreef A (2018) Impact of pelvic floor muscle training on sexual function ofwomen with urinary incontinence and a comparison ofelectrical stimulation versus standard treatment (IPSU trial): a randomised controlled trial S. Physiotherapy 104:91–97

Kavvadias T, Baessler K, Schuessler B (2011) Pelvic pain in urogynaecology. Part I: evaluation, definitions and diagnoses. Int J Urogynecol 22:385–393

Kellogg-Spadt S, Iorio J, Fariello JY et al (2012) Vaginal dilation: when it's indicated, and tips on teaching it. Obstet Gynecol Manag 24:12

Knoepp LR, Shippey SH, Chen CC, Cundiff GW, Derogatis LR, Handa VL (2010) Sexual complaints, pelvic floor symptoms, and sexual distress in women over forty. J Sex Med 7(11):3675–3682

Kotarinos RK (2003) Pelvic floor physical therapy in urogynecologic disorders. Curr Womens Health Rep 3(4):334–339

Lahaie MA, Amsel R, Khalifé S, Boyer S, Faaborg-Andersen M, Binik YM (2015) Can fear, pain, and muscle tension discriminate vaginismus from dyspareunia/provoked vestibulodynia? Implications for the new DSM-5 diagnosis of Genito-pelvic pain/penetration disorder. Arch Sex Behav 44(6):1537–1550

Laumann EO, Paik A, Rosen RC (1999) Sexual dysfunction in the United States: prevalence and predictors. JAMA 281(6):537–544. Erratum in: JAMA 281(13):1174

Laursen BS, Bajaj P, Olesen AS, Delmar C, Arendt-Nielsen L (2005) Health related quality of life and quantitative pain measurement in females with chronic non-malignant pain. Eur J Pain 9(3):267–275

Morin M, Dumoulin C, Bergeron S, Mayrand M, Khalifé S, Waddell G, Dubois M, Provoked vestibulodynia (PVD) Study Group (2016) Randomized clinical trial of multimodal physiotherapy treatment compared to overnight lidocaine ointment in women with provoked vestibulodynia: design and methods. Contemp Clin Trials 46:52–59

Nazarpour S, Simbar M, Majd HA, Tehrani FR (2018) Beneficial effects of pelvic floor muscle exercises on sexual function among postmenopausal women: a randomised clinical trial. Sex Health 15(5):396–402

Pacik PT (2014) Understanding and treating vaginismus: a multimodal approach. Int Urogynecol J 25:1613–1620

Pastore EA, Katzman WB (2012) Recognizing myofascial pelvic pain in the female patient with chronic pelvic pain. J Obstet Gynecol Neonatal Nurs 41(5):680–691

Penney JN (2010) The biopsychosocial model of pain and contemporary osteopathic practice. Int J Osteop Med 13(2):42–47

Rosenbaum TY (2011) How well is the multidisciplinary model working? J Sex Med 8:2957–2958

Sadovsky R, Mulhall JP (2003) The potential value of erectile dysfunction inquiry and management. Int J Clin Pract 57:601–608

Sadownik LA, Seal BN, Brotto LA (2012) Provoked vestibulodynia—women's experience of participating in a multidisciplinary vulvodynia program. J Sex Med 9:1086–1093

Salonia A, Zanni G, Nappi RE, Briganti A, Dehò F, Fabbri F, Colombo R, Guazzoni G, Di Girolamo V, Rigatti P, Montorsi F (2004) Sexual dysfunction is common in women with lower urinary tract symptoms and urinary incontinence: results of a cross-sectional study. Eur Urol 45(5):642–648. discussion 648

Santrock JW (2007) A topical approach to human life-span development, 3rd edn. McGraw-Hill, St. Louis, MO

Schvartzman R, Schvartzman L, Ferreira CF et al (2019) Physical therapy intervention for women with dyspareunia: a randomized clinical trial. J Sex Marital Ther 45:378–394

Simons DG (1996) Clinical and etiological update of myofascial pain from trigger points. J Musculoskelet Pain 4(1–2):93–122

Simons DG, Travell JG, Simons LS (1992) Myofascial pain and dysfunction: the trigger point manual, vol 2. Williams & Wilkins, Baltimore, MD

Simons DG, Travell JG, Simons LS (1999) Myofascial pain and dysfunction: the trigger point manual, vol 1, 2nd edn. Williams & Wilkins, Baltimore, MD

Srinivasan AK, Kaye JD, Moldwin R (2007) Myofascial dysfunction associated with chronic pelvic floor pain: management strategies. Curr Pain Headache Rep 11(5):359–364

Vallinga MS, Spoelstra SK, Hemel ILM, van de Wiel HBM, Weijmar Schultz WCM (2015) Transcutaneous electrical nerve stimulation as an additional treatment for women suffering from therapy-resistant provoked vestibulodynia: a feasibility study. J Sex Med 12:228–237

Weiss PM, Rich J, Swisher E (2012) Pelvic floor spasm: the missing link in chronic pelvic pain. Contemp OB/GYN. October 1, http://contemporaryobgyn.modernmedicine.com

WHO (2018) International classification of functioning, disability and health. World Health Organisation, Geneva

Wijma AJ, Paul van Wilgen C, Meeus M, Nijs J (2016) Clinical biopsychosocial physiotherapy assessment of patients with chronic pain: the first step in pain neuroscience education. Physiother Theory Pract 32(5):368–384. https://doi.org/10.1080/09593985.2016.1194651

Willard F (2008) Basic mechanisms of pain. In: Audette JF, Bailey A (eds) Integrative pain medicine: the science and practice of complementary and alternative medicine in pain management. Humana Press, Totowa, NJ, pp 19–61

Williams RE, Hartmann KE, Steege JF (2004) Documenting the current definitions of chronic pelvic pain: implications for research. Obstet Gynecol 103(4):686–691

Zoorob D, South M, Karram M, Sroga J, Maxwell R, Shah A, Whiteside J (2015) A pilot randomized trial of levator injections versus physical therapy for treatment of pelvic floor myalgia and sexual pain. Int Urogynecol J 26:845–852

Pharmacological and Surgical Management

14

Victoria Kershaw and Swati Jha

14.1 Background

The management of Female Sexual Dysfunction (FSD) by the nurse specialist/allied health professional requires a knowledge of the various treatment options as well as the drug interactions which may impact on sexual function. An understanding of the multidimensional female sexual response cycle is imperative prior to offering or proposing treatments. These include emotional, physical, psychological as well as interpersonal components and have been discussed in other chapters. A detailed history and examination will highlight the aspects of female sexual function affected so this can be addressed.

In this chapter we will discuss the various pharmacological treatments to address the problem and will also consider medications which are used in different conditions that impact adversely on sexual function. The impact of various surgical treatment options will also be discussed.

14.2 Pharmacological Management

Pharmacological therapy is just one aspect of the multifaceted management that may be required when treating FSD. For a number of women, a combination of medication alongside psychological and physical therapies may be necessary.

Author Contributions:
VK: Researched and wrote the chapter, editing and approval of final version.
SJ: Senior author on chapter, researched and wrote the chapter, editing and approval of final version.

V. Kershaw · S. Jha (✉)
Sheffield Teaching Hospitals NHS Foundation Trust, Sheffield, UK
e-mail: Swati.Jha1@nhs.uk

© Springer Nature Switzerland AG 2021
A. Rantell (ed.), *Sexual Function and Pelvic Floor Dysfunction*,
https://doi.org/10.1007/978-3-030-63843-6_14

Table 14.1 Impact of medications on female sexual function

Medication	Impact on sexual function
Anti-hypertensives, e.g. thiazide diuretics, beta-blockers	Can lead to a reduction in genital engorgement leading to lubrication difficulties and reduced sexual pleasure
Anti-depressants, e.g. selective serotonin reuptake inhibitors (SSRIs)	Increase serotonin, inhibit dopamine and noradrenaline which can negatively impact the processes of desire, arousal and lubrication
Anti-psychotics	Can cause dopamine blockade, high prolactin and low oestrogen, resulting in reduced sexual desire/arousal, vaginal dryness, dyspareunia and galactorrhoea
Anti-convulsants	Result in lower testosterone levels which in turn can reduce sexual desire/arousal
Hormonal contraception	Decrease free testosterone levels which may lead to reduced sexual desire
Anti-oestrogens, e.g. tamoxifen, GnRH analogues, letrozole	May result in vulvovaginal atrophy causing lubrication difficulties and dyspareunia
Anti-androgens, e.g. cimetidine, spironolactone, cyproterone acetate	Cause lower testosterone levels which may reduce sexual desire/arousal
Steroids	Cause lower testosterone levels which may reduce sexual desire/arousal
Opiates, sedatives, hypnotics	Reduce sexual performance and delay orgasm
Immunosuppressants, e.g. cyclophosphamide	Can impair gonadal function, reduce oestrogen levels and cause vulvovaginal atrophy
Anti-histamines	Associated with low sexual desire
Metoclopramide	Inhibit dopamine, increase prolactin leading to hypogonadism and negative impacts on desire, arousal, lubrication and potentially vulvovaginal atrophy
Metronidazole	Associated with low sexual desire

Before considering pharmacological therapy for FSD it is first important to review the patient's current medication. There are a number of medications that contribute to FSD in different ways (Table 14.1).

If a patient is taking a medication which may be causing or contributing to their sexual dysfunction, it is prudent to ask the GP or prescriber to consider alternatives or reducing the dose of the medication. Clearly this will not be possible in all instances, but an awareness of this may reassure the patient that there is nothing inherently wrong with them.

Pharmacological therapies for FSD are varied in their mechanism of action. Broadly they can be categorised into the following groups: hormone replacement, vasodilators and centrally acting drugs.

14.2.1 Hormone Replacement

14.2.1.1 Oestrogen
Both systemic and vaginal oestrogen can be used to treat FSD related to genito-urinary syndrome of the menopause (GSM).

Topical oestrogen: Vaginal oestrogen has minimal systemic absorption and therefore is associated with fewer adverse effects than oral/transdermal preparations (Shifren 2003). For this reason it is generally considered the treatment of choice for GSM. Topical oestrogen is currently available in the form of a vaginal ring, vaginal creams and vaginal pessaries (Srivastava et al. 2008). Ideally the treatment is used at night prior to bed so there is minimal movement after administration and most of the product will remain inside the vagina for a number of hours. Regimes of treatment may vary but usually begin with intensive daily treatment until symptoms are controlled (often a 2-week period), reducing to twice per week thereafter. Patients can repeat a course of intensive treatment in the future, as and when required for an exacerbation of symptoms. Topical lubricants and vaginal moisturisers can also be used alongside topical oestrogen if necessary. Long-term use is now considered safe, although historically women were asked to take breaks from treatment and this practice does still occasionally occur. Indeed data does not appear to show an increased risk of cancer recurrence in women with a history of oestrogen-dependent cancer using topical oestrogen, although many clinicians and patients may still feel uncomfortable with any form of hormonal treatment in this group (Vegunta et al. 2016).

Postnatal women who describe FSD should be asked about breastfeeding. Breastfeeding women are significantly more likely to report lack of sexual desire. Lactating women can also experience the effects of a hypooestrogenic state resulting in dyspareunia and vaginal dryness. Women can be reassured that they are likely to experience improvement of sexual function within weeks of cessation of breastfeeding. For most women this will be sufficient reassurance and they may not wish any further treatment. For women who request therapy, topical oestrogen would be recommended for use as a short-term treatment during lactation (Bachmann et al. 2002).

Systemic oestrogen: Oestrogen plays a key role in sexual function; however, there is no direct correlation between oestrogen levels and sexual symptoms (van Lunsen and Laan 2004). Therefore, the use of systemic oestrogen must be considered carefully and would not be routine practice for the treatment of FSD in menopausal women. There are a number of risks associated with systemic oestrogen replacement including increased breast and ovarian cancer risk, venous thromboembolism and stroke. Systemic oestrogen in the form of hormone replacement therapy (HRT) and combined hormonal contraception has also been reported to have a negative impact on sexual desire in some studies, although evidence is mixed (FSRH Clinical Effectiveness Unit 2009).

There are however some women for whom the benefits of treatment with systemic oestrogen would outweigh the risks. This includes women suffering from both systemic menopausal symptoms such as vasomotor flushes and night sweats, as well as vulvovaginal atrophy. Women who undergo a surgical menopause following removal of both ovaries are also recommended to take hormone replacement therapy until the age of the natural menopause (50–51 years) primarily due to the high risk of osteoporosis but it is also helpful in preventing GSM. Systemic oestrogen is also used in the treatment of various concomitant gynaecological conditions such as dysfunctional uterine bleeding and endometriosis, in the form of combined hormonal contraception (oestrogen and progestogen). When taken cyclically, combined hormonal contraception can be used to control erratic bleeding and also lighten menstrual flow by thinning the endometrium. When taken continuously it can be used to suppress the proliferation of endometriotic deposits and induce amenorrhoea in the treatment of endometriosis. In this situation systemic oestrogen may help to ameliorate sexual dysfunction which is directly related to the condition. Overall systemic oestrogen generally would not be considered first-line for a patient presenting with FSD alone.

Systemic oestrogen is available in the form of oral tablets or transdermal patches. Transdermal patches are associated with a lower risk of venous thromboembolism than oral preparations. For women who have a uterus or a history of endometriosis, combined HRT with both oestrogen and progesterone is required to prevent hyperplasia of the endometrium or endometriotic foci. Prescriptions should be reviewed regularly to ensure that the minimum effective dose is used for the shortest duration.

14.2.1.2 Intravaginal Prasterone (Intrarosa°)

Prasterone is a steroid precursor which is converted to oestrogen and androgens. It is licenced for the treatment of GSM. Several studies have shown a moderate benefit for vulvovaginal atrophy although prasterone has not been compared directly with other treatments. The majority of clinicians are of the opinion that topical oestrogen is a more effective and more thoroughly investigated treatment for GSM and this would generally be chosen first-line. Prasterone may have a place in the treatment algorithm for women with who have not responded to initial treatment, but it is not widely used at present (BMJ Publishing Group 2019).

14.2.1.3 Ospemifene (Senshio°)

Ospemifene is a selective oestrogen receptor modulator. It has been shown to be an effective treatment for dyspareunia secondary to vulvovaginal atrophy (Cui et al. 2014).

14.2.1.4 Tibolone

Tibolone is a unique form of HRT as it is a synthetic steroid with oestrogenic, progestogenic and androgenic properties. It is a particularly good choice of HRT for women with FSD who require treatment for systemic menopausal symptoms. Studies have shown that in postmenopausal women with FSD, tibolone improved overall sexual function, increased frequency of sex and reduced sexually-related personal distress (Nijland et al. 2008). Women suffering from low sexual desire may find this especially helpful. However, tibolone is associated with a higher increased risk of stroke and endometrial cancer than other HRT options (British National Formulary 2019).

14.2.1.5 Testosterone

Testosterone production naturally declines after the menopause. Low levels of testosterone are associated with decreased libido, arousal and orgasm (Masters and Johnson 1966). Testosterone therapy has been reported to result in significant improvement in various domains of sexual function in postmenopausal women (Elraiyah et al. 2014). It is available in the form of a transdermal patch or a gel but is an off licence prescription in the UK and women need to be informed of this if they are to be prescribed treatment. NICE guidelines on menopause now recommend considering testosterone supplementation for women with low sexual desire if HRT alone is not effective (National Institute for Health and Care Excellence (NICE) 2019). However, there is a lack of long-term safety data and a number of undesirable side effects including alopecia, hirsutism, acne, breast pain, headache, adverse liver function, lipid profile change and increased risk of cardiovascular disease, insulin resistance and metabolic syndrome (Srivastava et al. 2008; Elraiyah et al. 2014; Khajehei et al. 2015). It is perhaps best suited to patients suffering from surgical menopause or a medical condition resulting in androgen deficiency. In surgical menopause there is an abrupt 50% reduction in production of testosterone in contrast to the gradual decline in ovarian and adrenal androgen production that ordinarily occurs naturally with age (Srivastava et al. 2008).

The American College of Obstetricians and Gynaecologists suggest that if prescribed, a 3–6-month trial is recommended with assessment of testosterone levels at baseline and after 3–6 weeks of initial use to ensure levels remain within the normal range. They also suggest that if ongoing therapy is used, follow-up clinical evaluation and testosterone measurement should take place every 6 months to assess for androgen excess (The American College of Obstetricians and Gynaecologists 2019).

14.2.2 Vasodilators

Drugs that cause vasodilation are designed to aid genital engorgement, which in turn relates to lubrication and arousal.

Phosphodiesterase type 5 inhibitors, such as sildenafil (Viagra®), cause vascular smooth muscle relaxation and vasodilation via the nitric oxide signalling pathway. Evidence regarding the use of sildenafil in FSD is mixed. Early clinical trials in which women with sexual desire/arousal disorder were treated with sildenafil showed promising results (Allahdadi et al. 2009). Sildenafil has also been shown to be beneficial to women with spinal cord injury and FSD secondary to use of SSRIs (selective serotonin reuptake inhibitors) (Srivastava et al. 2008). However an RCT with 781 women with sexual arousal disorder did not report any conclusive improvement with sildenafil. It is not currently a licenced treatment for FSD (Basson et al. 2002).

Other drugs currently under investigation are L-arginine, prostaglandin, phentolamine and VIP (vasoactive intestinal peptide) which all have a theoretical mechanism to improve genital engorgement by vasodilation.

14.2.3 Centrally Acting Drugs

The medications in this category represent an alternative approach to treatment of FSD as they act centrally in the brain to influence behavioural states.

Dopamine agonists have been shown to be effective in increasing sexual desire in women with hypoactive sexual desire disorder (Allahdadi et al. 2009). Furthermore, cabergoline has been shown to improve sexual function in anti-psychotic induced hyperprolactinaemia (Kalkavoura et al. 2013). Similarly, bupropion has been shown to help ameliorate the negative effects on sexual function associated with SSRI use (Wright and O'Connor 2015). However, given the central action of these drugs there is also a high occurrence of side effects such as nausea, vomiting and headaches (Allahdadi et al. 2009).

Sublingual/intranasal apomorphine is currently under investigation with the hope this will be quicker acting than oral administration and be associated with fewer side effects (Srivastava et al. 2008; Allahdadi et al. 2009).

Use of the centrally acting agent α-melanocortin-stimulating hormone in treatment of FSD is also in development and has shown promising results in pre-clinical trials (Allahdadi et al. 2009).

Flibanserin is a serotonin 1a agonist/2a antagonist approved by the FDA in 2015 for treatment of hypoactive sexual desire in pre-menopausal women. However, a systematic review showed there was minimal or no improvement of symptoms with this treatment and a high prevalence of adverse effects such as dizziness, fatigue and nausea. The patient must also agree to abstain from alcohol whilst on this medication as the interaction is known to produce hypotension and syncope (The American College of Obstetricians and Gynaecologists 2019). It is not currently available in the UK and Europe.

14.2.4 Muscle Relaxants

Tizanidine is a centrally active alpha 2 agonist used as a muscle relaxant, which has been shown to be superior to placebo in treating high-tone pelvic floor dysfunction (Nickel et al. 2007).

14.2.5 Vitamin Supplementation

Vitamin C in addition to antimicrobial treatment has been used successfully to treat dyspareunia related to chlamydial infection (Khajehei et al. 2015).

Calcium plus vitamin D alongside dydrogesterone have been used to improve lack of sexual desire before menstruation (Khajehei et al. 2015).

14.3   Drug Treatment for Other Conditions Causing FSD

Women presenting with FSD should be assessed for underlying vulval and other conditions that may impact on sexual function.

14.3.1 Vulval Disease

Lichen sclerosus/planus—exacerbations are managed with ultrapotent topical steroids. Maintenance therapy may be with either weaker topical steroids or less frequent use of potent ones (Edwards et al. 2015) . Whilst there is good evidence that this treatment is effective in reducing vulval discomfort, the effect of this treatment on sexual function has not been fully evaluated (Haefner et al. 2014). One study did show that despite adequate treatment, FSD may persist for some patients (Burrows et al. 2011).

Vulval eczema/psoriasis—treatment involves use of an emollient soap substitute and intermittent mild topical steroids. Weak coal tar and vitamin D analogues may be useful adjuncts for psoriasis (Edwards et al. 2015). Similarly the effect of these treatments on sexual function has not been studied.

Vulval intraepithelial neoplasia (VIN)—treatment of this premalignant condition is primarily surgical; however, patients may be offered an alternative in the form of imiquimod 5% cream (Edwards et al. 2015). This topical immunomodulator is associated with a temporary burning pain but no long-term sexual dysfunction has been reported suggesting any symptoms are reversible (Ribeiro et al. 2012).

Vulvodynia—vulvodynia may be localised and provoked or generalised and unprovoked. For both conditions avoiding triggers and using an emollient soap substitute are essential first steps. Patients may find local anaesthetic gel helpful, particularly prior to intercourse, especially those with localised provoked symptoms. Neuropathic pain modifiers may also be beneficial, although evidence is mixed. Amitriptyline is recommended first-line. Gabapentin and pregabalin may be considered if this is not tolerated or effective. Physical and psychological therapies are often also necessary. Vestibulectomy is occasionally performed for localised provoked vulvodynia that is refractory to other treatments (see Sect. 14.4) (Edwards et al. 2015). None of the pharmacological options have been investigated with regard to sexual function in this condition.

14.3.2 Benign Gynaecological Disorders

Fibroids: Fibroids may cause pelvic pressure symptoms including dyspareunia and are also associated with heavy menstrual bleeding, which may impact on sexual function. Gonadotrophin releasing hormone (GnRH) analogues may be used for 3 months pre-operatively in order to shrink a fibroid prior to myomectomy or hysterectomy. They may also be used as a bridge to the menopause in managing symptoms, as fibroids tend to shrink after menopause is attained. Ordinarily GnRH is produced by the hypothalamus in a pulsatile fashion. It stimulates the pituitary gland to produce FSH (follicle stimulating hormone) and LH (luteinising hormone) which in turn act on the ovary to produce oestrogen and progesterone. When GnRH analogues are given, there is a constant stimulation of the pituitary as opposed to the physiological pulsatile release, which paradoxically inhibits the production of FSH and LH resulting in a temporary menopausal (hypooestrogenic) state. Fibroids are oestrogen-dependent benign tumours so when deprived of oestrogen in this way they shrink. Whilst a patient is undergoing this treatment, they are prone to developing menopausal symptoms such as vasomotor symptoms and vaginal dryness. If the patient is struggling to manage these symptoms, they can take add-back HRT in the form of tibolone which has minimal effect on the size of the fibroid (Moroni et al. 2015). Add-back vaginal oestrogen for genito-urinary symptoms has not been investigated for this group of patients. The menopausal symptoms are reversible after cessation of treatment.

Endometriosis: In endometriosis the mainstay of treatment is to suppress endometrial proliferation by inducing amenorrhoea. Both continuous combined hormonal contraception and progestogens in various forms (injectable, Mirenacoil®, pills) are used to do this. Decreased sexual desire have been reported in patients using both combined hormonal contraception and progestogens (FSRH Clinical Effectiveness Unit 2009, 2014, 2019a, b). However, in this specific group of women, these treatments help to alleviate symptoms of pelvic pain, dyspareunia and heavy/painful/erratic bleeding and have been shown to have a positive effect on sexual function (Caruso et al. 2016; Sansone et al. 2018). GnRH analogues are also used either for short-term symptom relief or to help predict a response to surgery. Their effect on sexual function is discussed above. Surgical treatment is also commonly required for these patients in the form of excision of endometriosis and for some ultimately hysterectomy and oophorectomy may be required (see Sect. 14.4).

14.3.3 Urological

Overactive bladder (OAB): Patients suffering from OAB have a particularly high prevalence of sexual dysfunction with women reporting a number of problems including loss of body image, coital incontinence, lack of lubrication and sexual pain. First-line treatment for this condition is lifestyle modification, elimination of bladder irritants and bladder retraining. Anticholinergic medications such as tolterodine and solifenacin are commonly prescribed as an adjunct to these conservative measures. Several studies have shown that female sexual function improves significantly in all domains including desire, arousal, lubrication and orgasm in women taking this treatment for OAB (Gali et al. 2019). The improvement in lubrication is particularly notable as a recognised side effect of anticholinergics is dry mucous membranes (eyes and mouth). Although in one study the benefit was more modest with only 8% of women reporting improvement in sexual function (Jha 2016). Mirabegron is a β_3-adrenergic agonist which is used in OAB treatment if anticholinergic medication is not tolerated or effective. Similarly studies have also shown that sexual function improves significantly in patients taking this medication for OAB (Gali et al. 2019). If OAB is refractory to medical treatment, patients may go on to have intravesical Botox® injections, sacral neuromodulation or percutaneous tibial nerve stimulation (see Sect. 14.4).

Painful bladder syndrome: Painful bladder syndrome is strongly associated with sexual dysfunction, particularly due to dyspareunia symptoms. Initial treatment of painful bladder syndrome involves a combination of painkillers, anti-histamines, OAB drugs and pentosan polysulphate sodium (Elmiron®). If these treatments are not effective, the patient may require a series of bladder instillations. The composition of the instillations can vary but commonly they consist of a mixture of local anaesthetic, hyaluronic acid and chondroitin sulphate. Studies have shown that there is a statistically significant improvement in all domains of sexual function (desire, arousal, lubrication, orgasm, satisfaction and pain) at 6 months post treatment with hyaluronic acid/chondroitin sulphate or with chondroitin sulphate alone (Arslan et al. 2019).

14.4 Surgical Management

The role of surgery in the management of FSD may be either to treat an underlying condition such as prolapse, urinary incontinence or endometriosis, or it may be in the treatment of a primary sexual problem such as Botox® injections for refractory vaginismus or Fenton's procedure for dyspareunia related to a posterior fourchette skin bridge post obstetric injury.

14.4.1 Surgical Treatment of Pelvic Organ Prolapse (POP)

In the surgical treatment of pelvic organ prolapse (POP), there is a risk that the nerves and vessels supplying the vagina and external genitalia may be disrupted which could in turn have a negative impact on sexual dysfunction (Srivastava et al. 2008). This risk must be discussed with patients as part of the consent process prior to surgery. It is important that unrealistic expectations are therefore not given to women awaiting surgery for various pelvic floor disorders.

For treatment of anterior and posterior compartment prolapse, the most commonly performed procedure is pelvic floor repair (colporrhaphy). This involves reconstructing the fascial layers supporting the vagina either anteriorly or posteriorly with dissolvable sutures. If there is concomitant prolapse in the apical compartment, then these procedures may be combined with a vaginal hysterectomy (if the uterus is present).

A recent study examining the effect of pelvic floor repair on sexual function showed that 47% improved, 39% remained unchanged, 18% deteriorated and 4% reported new onset dyspareunia, although this study was unable to separate results by compartment (Jha and Gray 2015). In a prospective study of women undergoing anterior pelvic floor repair with/without hysterectomy, there was a significant improvement in sexual function at 6 months (Dua et al. 2012). Outcomes following posterior pelvic floor repair were slightly less clear. Vaginal narrowing and shortening which occur more commonly with posterior repair may cause problems. Partner discomfort has also been reported post-operatively (Srivastava et al. 2008). In the same prospective study, there was an improvement in sexual function following posterior repair but in the dyspareunia domain the improvement failed to reach statistical significance (Dua et al. 2012). Increased post-operative dyspareunia was found consistently when anterior and posterior repairs were combined in the same procedure, and many gynaecologists may consider a two-stage procedure for sexually active women requiring repair to both compartments (Srivastava et al. 2008; Dua et al. 2012).

In the surgical management of post hysterectomy apical (vaginal vault) prolapse, there are two main treatment options: vaginal sacrospinous fixation and abdominal sacrocolpopexy. In sacrospinous fixation, the vaginal vault is attached to the pelvic sacrospinous ligament with dissolvable sutures via a vaginal incision. In sacrocolpopexy, the vaginal vault is attached to the sacrum using a bridge of polypropylene mesh via an open or laparoscopic abdominal approach. With regard to sexual function, sacrospinous fixation is associated with higher rates of post-operative dyspareunia than abdominal sacrocolpopexy (Maher et al. 2013).

Altered perception of genital health after surgery with associated fear of damaging oneself can also have a negative impact on FSD (Srivastava et al. 2008). However, despite the theoretical risks, on the whole sexual dysfunction improves following prolapse repair.

The use of vaginal mesh for POP, which has now fallen in disrepute and is no longer performed, was another recognised cause for dyspareunia related to scarring caused by mesh contracture and exposure. When patients describe dyspareunia following a mesh repair, mesh exposure should be ruled out as a matter of urgency (Campbell et al. 2018). Hispareunia (partner dyspareunia) is another recognised risk of mesh repair and has been reported with mesh exposure.

14.4.2 Surgical Treatment of Urinary Incontinence

The surgical options available for the treatment of stress urinary incontinence include mid-urethral mesh tape, colposuspension, autologous fascial sling and urethral bulking agents. Excluding bulking agents, all operations are designed to support the mid-urethra and limit urethral hypermobility to ultimately reduce incontinence episodes. In a mid-urethral tape, a strip of polypropylene mesh is inserted via a vagina incision. In a colposuspension, the lateral walls of the vagina are sutured to Cooper's ligament in the pelvis to effectively create a sling around the upper urethra. In an autologous fascial sling a strip of fascia is harvested, usually from the rectus sheath in the abdominal wall, and repurposed to create a sling around the mid-urethra. In urethral bulking, the agent is injected into the wall of the urethra under cystoscopic vision in order to narrow the upper urethra.

Research has shown that following surgery for stress urinary incontinence (mid-urethral tape/colposuspension/autologous fascial sling), coital incontinence is likely to improve. However, overall sexual function is likely to remain unchanged, though there is a small possibility of improvement or even deterioration following surgery (Jha et al. 2012). The effect of urethral bulking agents on sexual function has not been studied. Women should be informed of this prior to surgery to avoid disappointment following surgery.

In the surgical treatment of overactive bladder and urge urinary incontinence, the options are intravesical Botox® injection, sacral neuromodulation and percutaneous tibial nerve stimulation. In intravesical Botox treatment, botulinum toxin A is injected at multiple sites in the bladder wall via a cystoscope. This reduces the ability of the bladder muscle to contract and thus reduces urgency. The effect of intravesical Botox® injection on sexual function has not been studied extensively but some small studies have reported an improvement in sexual function in all domains (Miotla et al. 2017). In sacral neuromodulation (SNS), a device is implanted subcutaneously in the buttock with a pacing wire inserted into the S3 nerve root. This stimulates the nervous innervation of the pelvic organs and can improve both urinary and faecal incontinence with a success rate of up to 80%. In percutaneous tibial nerve stimulation (PTNS), a fine gauge needle is inserted behind the medial malleolus of the ankle. This is attached to a battery operated stimulator for a 30 min treatment, which is repeated weekly for 12 weeks. The posterior tibial nerve shares the same nerve routes as the nerves innervating the bladder. This alternative neuromodulation technique has also been shown to be an effective treatment for urinary and faecal incontinence but with lower success rates in the region of 60%. Some studies show promising results regarding the effect of SNS and PTNS on FSD in patients undergoing treatment for pelvic floor dysfunction (Khunda et al. 2019; Kershaw et al. 2019). However, neuromodulation as a treatment for a primary sexual dysfunction has not yet been studied.

14.4.3 Hysterectomy for the Treatment of Benign Gynaecological Disease, e.g. Dysfunctional Uterine Bleeding, Endometriosis

Sexual function after hysterectomy has been studied extensively. It has been hypothesised that damage to the autonomic nerve endings of the cervicovaginal area and vaginal shortening may interfere with lubrication, orgasm and sexual pleasure (Jewett 1952). In addition, hysterectomy may have psychological effects leading to loss of feminine identity and self-esteem (Srivastava et al. 2008). The largest prospective study to date is the Maryland Women's Health Study which found that at 24 months post hysterectomy there was increased frequency of sexual activity, and improvement in dyspareunia, orgasm, libido and vaginal dryness (Rhodes et al. 1999). The surgical approach (abdominal, vaginal, laparoscopic) did not affect sexual outcomes. The method of vaginal cuff closure did not impact on sexual function (Jha 2019). Furthermore, a randomised trial comparing total versus subtotal hysterectomy found no difference in post-operative dyspareunia, quality of orgasm or sexual satisfaction. Concomitant oophorectomy can however be implicated in FSD, particularly in pre-menopausal women due to the resultant abrupt reduction in oestrogen and testosterone production. Hormone replacement therapy is generally recommended in patients undergoing bilateral oophorectomy under the age of 50 years. Replacement testosterone can also be offered if necessary.

14.4.4 Vestibulectomy

The vulval vestibule is the area between the labia minora into which the urethral meatus and the vaginal introitus open into. Surgical vestibulectomy has been used successfully as a treatment for localised provoked vulvodynia. In this procedure, the painful tissues of the vestibule are identified and removed. An RCT by Bergeron et al. reported significantly less dyspareunia in patients with localised vulvodynia who underwent vestibulectomy in comparison to treatment with CBT and electromyographic biofeedback (Bergeron et al. 2001). Patients who have responded to the use of pre-coital lidocaine are most likely to report a better outcome. Vestibulectomy is now rarely performed in the UK.

14.4.5 Fenton's Procedure

Fenton's procedure can be offered when a patient experiences dyspareunia secondary to narrowing, skin-splitting or formation of a skin bridge at the posterior fourchette, usually secondary to obstetric scarring or vulval dermatoses such as lichen sclerosus. During the procedure, the scar tissue/constriction band at the posterior fourchette is removed and the opening to the vagina is widened. Benefits from this procedure is probably modest and there is a paucity of evidence. A small study of 24 women by Chandru showed that at 12 months post-op, 14 women (60.8%) reported complete relief and moderate relief was reported in 9 (39%) (Chandru et al. 2010). However, worsening of dyspareunia is a potential risk.

14.4.6 Trigger Point Injections

In trigger point injections, a mixture of local anaesthetic and anti-inflammatory steroid is injected into the pelvic floor at a pre-identified trigger point of pain/spasm. A prospective study investigated the role of trigger point injections in women with levator ani muscle spasm with a mixture of 0.25% bupivacaine, 2% lidocaine and 40 mg of triamcinolone combined and used for injection of 5 ml per trigger point. Three months after injections, 72% of women reported improvement (Langford et al. 2007).

14.4.7 Botox® Injections to the Pelvic Floor Muscles

Refractory vaginismus may respond to Botox® injections into puborectalis/pubococcygeus muscles of the pelvic floor (Morrissey et al. 2015; Ghazizadeh and Nikzad 2004). The injection can help to relax/paralyse the pelvic floor muscles to prevent spasm and allow intercourse. Once regular intercourse is successfully established, the anxiety related to penetration is relieved and the cycle of anxiety/spasm/dyspareunia is broken, hopefully resulting in maintenance of successful intercourse even after the effect of Botox® on the muscles has worn off.

14.4.8 Lasers

Laser therapy of the vagina is an emerging technology and it has been marketed as a treatment for a number of genital complaints. However, evidence of efficacy and long-term safety is lacking for the use of laser therapy in most contexts.

One group of patients potentially set to benefit the most from laser treatment are breast cancer survivors. Breast cancer patients have a high prevalence of vulvovaginal atrophy and associated lubrication difficulties, dyspareunia and low level of sexual desire (Sbitti et al. 2011). Most clinicians and patients will not feel comfortable prescribing topical oestrogen to this group of women, but lubricants and vaginal moisturisers have limited efficacy when used alone in the treatment of severe vulvovaginal atrophy. Preliminary data for both erbium and carbon dioxide vaginal lasers in the treatment of vulvovaginal atrophy are promising. In a recent systematic review, vaginal laser therapy was found to be effective in treating vulvovaginal atrophy in breast cancer survivors with improvement in dyspareunia, vaginal dryness and sexual function (Jha et al. 2019). There is an urgent need for good quality data before introduction into practice.

Carbon dioxide lasers have also been used to treat refractory lichen sclerosus successfully. In a small study of 40 women with steroid resistant lichen sclerosus by Pagano et al., there was a statistically significant improvement in vulval itching, dryness, dyspareunia and sensitivity related to intercourse following laser treatment (Pagano et al. 2020). However, this finding has yet to be replicated in larger randomised controlled trials.

Lasers have also been marketed for use in genital cosmetic surgery, including vaginoplasty and rejuvenation surgery. These surgeries have been developed with the aim of improving the appearance and/or function of the female genital tract. However, evidence supporting the efficacy and safety of these procedures is lacking (Rogers et al. 2018).

14.5 Recommendations for Treatment

- Treat underlying causes, e.g. prolapse, incontinence, endometriosis.
- Review current medication for drugs that may be causing dysfunction for example SSRIs.
- Do not overlook genito-urinary syndrome of the menopause (GSM)—it is common and there are effective treatments available that can alleviate sexual symptoms. Use topical oestrogen if isolated GSM. Consider systemic oestrogen if menopausal symptoms as well as GSM.
- Laser therapy is an emerging treatment for vulvovaginal atrophy.
- Examine carefully for vulval dermatoses and treat appropriately. Consider referral to Specialist Vulval Clinic if initial treatment fails.
- Consider tibolone for patients suffering from both menopausal symptoms and low sexual desire.

- Testosterone supplementation may be considered in menopausal patients suffering from low sexual desire if HRT alone is not effective as per NICE guidelines.
- For patients undergoing surgical menopause, recommended HRT with or without testosterone until natural age of menopause (51 years).
- For primary sexual problems, a number of approaches may be required including psychological and physical therapies.
- Refer to a specialist clinic if initial treatment measures for a primary sexual problem have failed (Sexual Dysfunction Clinic, Urogynaecology, Gynaecologist with Special Interest—provision will vary locally).

14.6 Conclusions

As the first point of contact for women with PFD, the nurse specialist/physiotherapist is uniquely placed to diagnose and identify the causes of FSD. This allows them to initiate management and direct women needing further management to the appropriate specialists. FSD is multidimensional and will often require a team effort between the woman, clinicians and trained therapists with a multidisciplinary approach.

Disclosure of Interests VK—none relevant to publication.
SJ—none relevant to publication.

References

Allahdadi KJ, Tostes RCA, Webb RC (2009) Female sexual dysfunction: therapeutic options and experimental challenges. Cardiovasc Hematol Agents Med Chem 4:260–269

Arslan B et al (2019) Outcomes of intravesical chondroitin-sulfate and combined hyaluronic-acid/chondroitin-sulfate therapy on female sexual function in bladder pain syndrome. Int Urogynecol J 30:1857–1862

Bachmann G et al (2002) Female androgen insufficiency: the Princeton consensus statement on definition, classification, and assessment. Fertil Steril 77:660–665

Basson R, McInnes R, Smith MD, Hodgson G, Koppiker N (2002) Efficacy and safety of sildenafil citrate in women with sexual dysfunction associated with female sexual arousal disorder. J Womens Health Gend Based Med 11:367–377

Bergeron S et al (2001) A randomized comparison of group cognitive–behavioral therapy, surface electromyographic biofeedback, and vestibulectomy in the treatment of dyspareunia resulting from vulvar vestibulitis. Pain 91:297–306

BMJ Publishing Group (2019) Prasterone for vulvar and vaginal atrophy. Drug Ther Bull 57:185–188

British National Formulary (2019) Treatment summary: sex hormones. British National Formulary, London

Burrows LJ, Creasey A, Goldstein AT (2011) The treatment of vulvar lichen Sclerosus and female sexual dysfunction. J Sex Med 8:219–222

Campbell P, Jha S, Cutner A (2018) Vaginal mesh in prolapse surgery. Obstet Gynaecol 20:49–56

Caruso S et al (2016) Comparative, open-label prospective study on the quality of life and sexual function of women affected by endometriosis-associated pelvic pain on 2 mg dienogest/30 µg ethinyl estradiol continuous or 21/7 regimen oral contraceptive. J Endocrinol Invest 39:923–931

Chandru S, Nafee T, Ismail K, Kettle C (2010) Evaluation of modified Fenton procedure for persistent superficial dyspareunia following childbirth. Gynecol Surg 7:245–248

Cui Y, Zong H, Yan H, Li N, Zhang Y (2014) The efficacy and safety of Ospemifene in treating dyspareunia associated with postmenopausal vulvar and vaginal atrophy: a systematic review and meta-analysis. J Sex Med 11:487–497

Dua A, Jha S, Farkas A, Radley S (2012) The effect of prolapse repair on sexual function in women. J Sex Med 9:1459–1465

Edwards SK, Bates CM, Lewis F, Sethi G, Grover D (2015) 2014 UK national guideline on the management of vulval conditions. Int J STD AIDS 26:611–624

Elraiyah T et al (2014) The benefits and harms of systemic testosterone therapy in postmenopausal women with Normal adrenal function: a systematic review and meta-analysis. J Clin Endocrinol Metab 99:3543–3550

FSRH Clinical Effectiveness Unit (2009) FSRH clinical guideline: combined hormonal contraception. https://www.fsrh.org/standards-and-guidance/documents/combined-hormonal-contraception/

FSRH Clinical Effectiveness Unit (2014) FSRH clinical guideline: progestogen-only implant. https://www.fsrh.org/standards-and-guidance/documents/cec-ceu-guidance-implants-feb-2014/

FSRH Clinical Effectiveness Unit (2019a) FSRH clinical guideline: progestogen-only injectable. https://www.fsrh.org/standards-and-guidance/documents/cec-ceu-guidance-injectables-dec-2014/

FSRH Clinical Effectiveness Unit (2019b) FSRH clinical guideline: progestogen-only pills. https://www.fsrh.org/standards-and-guidance/documents/cec-ceu-guidance-pop-mar-2015/

Gali L, Lior L, Levy G (2019) Overactive bladder syndrome treatments and their effect on female sexual function: a review. Sex Med 8:1–7

Ghazizadeh S, Nikzad M (2004) Botulinum toxin in the treatment of refractory vaginismus. Obstet Gynecol 104:922–925

Haefner HK et al (2014) The impact of vulvar lichen Sclerosus on sexual dysfunction. J Womens Health 23:765–770

Jewett JF (1952) Vaginal length and incidence of dyspareunia following total abdominal hysterectomy. Am J Obstet Gynecol 63:400–407

Jha S (2016) Impact of treatment of overactive bladder with anticholinergics on sexual function. Arch Gynecol Obstet 293:403–406

Jha S (2019) Maintaining sexual function after pelvic floor surgery. Climacteric 22:236–241

Jha S, Gray T (2015) A systematic review and meta-analysis of the impact of native tissue repair for pelvic organ prolapse on sexual function. Int Urogynecol J 26:321–327

Jha S, Ammenbal M, Metwally M (2012) Impact of incontinence surgery on sexual function: a systematic review and meta-analysis. J Sex Med 9:34–43

Jha S, Wyld L, Krishnaswamy PH (2019) The impact of vaginal laser treatment for genitourinary syndrome of menopause in breast cancer survivors: a systematic review and meta-analysis. Clin Breast Cancer 19:556–562

Kalkavoura CS et al (2013) Effects of Cabergoline on hyperprolactinemia, psychopathology, and sexual functioning in schizophrenic patients. Exp Clin Psychopharmacol 21:332–341

Kershaw V, Khunda A, McCormick C, Ballard P (2019) The effect of percutaneous tibial nerve stimulation (PTNS) on sexual function: a systematic review and meta-analysis. Int Urogynecol J 30:1619–1627

Khajehei M, Doherty M, Tilley PJM (2015) An update on sexual function and dysfunction in women. Arch Women Ment Health 18:423–433

Khunda A, McCormick C, Ballard P (2019) Sacral neuromodulation and sexual function: a systematic review and meta-analysis of the literature. Int Urogynecol J 30:339–352

Langford CF, Nagy SU, Ghoniem GM (2007) Levator ani trigger point injections: an underutilized treatment for chronic pelvic pain. NeurourolUrodyn 26:59–62

Maher C, Feiner B, Baessler K, Schmid C (2013) Surgical management of pelvic organ prolapse in women (review). Cochrane Database Syst Rev (4):CD004014

Masters W, Johnson V (1966) Human sexual response. Little, Brown, Boston

Miotla P et al (2017) Impact of intravesical onabotulinumtoxinA on sexual function in women with OAB. NeurourolUrodyn 36:1564–1569

Moroni RM et al (2015) Add-back therapy with GnRH analogues for uterine fibroids. Cochrane Database Syst Rev 2015(3):CD010854. https://doi.org/10.1002/14651858.cd010854.pub2

Morrissey D et al (2015) Botulinum toxin a injections into pelvic floor muscles under Electromyographic guidance for women with refractory high-tone pelvic floor dysfunction. Female Pelvic Med Reconstr Surg 21:277–282

National Institute for Health and Care Excellence (NICE) (2019) Menopause: diagnosis and management. NICE, London

Nickel JC, Baranowski AP, Pontari M, Berger RE, Tripp DA (2007) Management of men diagnosed with chronic prostatitis/chronic pelvic pain syndrome who have failed traditional management. Rev Urol 9:63–72

Nijland EA et al (2008) Tibolone and transdermal E2/NETA for the treatment of female sexual dysfunction in naturally menopausal women: results of a randomized active-controlled trial. J Sex Med 5:646–656

Pagano T et al (2020) Effect of rescue fractional microablative CO_2 laser on symptoms and sexual dysfunction in women affected by vulvar lichen sclerosus resistant to long-term use of topic corticosteroid: a prospective longitudinal study. Menopause 27:418–422

Rhodes JC, Kjerulff KH, Langenberg PW, Guzinski GM (1999) Hysterectomy and sexual functioning. JAMA 282:1934

Ribeiro F, Figueiredo A, Paula T, Borrego J (2012) Vulvar intraepithelial neoplasia: evaluation of treatment modalities. J Low Genit Tract Dis 16:313–317

Rogers RG et al (2018) An international Urogynecological association (IUGA)/international continence society (ICS) joint report on the terminology for the assessment of sexual health of women with pelvic floor dysfunction. NeurourolUrodyn 37:1220–1240

Sansone A et al (2018) Effects of etonogestrel implant on quality of life, sexual function, and pelvic pain in women suffering from endometriosis: results from a multicenter, prospective, observational study. Arch Gynecol Obstet 298:731–736

Sbitti Y et al (2011) Breast cancer treatment and sexual dysfunction: Moroccan women's perception. BMC Womens Health 11:29

Shifren JL (2003) Female sexual dysfunction after menopause. Harvard Medical School's Centre of Excellence in Women's Health, Vexing Clinical Issues in Women's Health Event Series 2003

Srivastava R, Thakar R, Sultan A (2008) Female sexual dysfunction in obstetrics and gynaecology. Obstet Gynecol Surv 8:527–537

The American College of Obstetricians and Gynaecologists (2019) Female sexual dysfunction. Pract Bull 1

van Lunsen R, Laan E (2004) Genital vascular responsiveness and sexual feelings in midlife women: psychophysiologic, brain, and genital imaging studies. Menopause 6:741–748

Vegunta S, Kling JM, Faubion SS (2016) Sexual health matters: management of female sexual dysfunction. J Womens Health 25:952–954

Wright JJ, O'Connor KM (2015) Female sexual dysfunction. Med Clin N Am 99:607–628

The Impact of Partner/Male Sexual Problems on Female Sexual Function

15

Angela Gregory

> **Key Points**
> - Sexual difficulties are increasingly common with age.
> - ED can be a marker for cardiovascular disease.
> - Difficulties with sexual function should be considered in the context of the couple relationship.
> - Asking about masturbation can provide a wealth of diagnostic information.
> - Encouraging healthy exploration and masturbation can be beneficial.
> - Combined pharmacological and psychological treatment often provides the best outcome for men with sexual dysfunction.
> - Psychosexual therapy.

15.1 Introduction

The physiological and psychological changes that occur at the time of the menopause may impact negatively on sexual function and relationship satisfaction. Vaginal dryness/atrophy, incontinence, prolapse, dyspareunia, changes in arousal and reduced sexual interest are common (Damsted 2012). Independently, men are also at an increased risk of erectile dysfunction as they age. There is evidence that ED in patients over 40 years is significantly associated with cardiovascular risk factors such as diabetes, hypertension, coronary artery disease, dyslipidaemia, atherosclerosis and metabolic syndrome (Kirana and Porst 2012). Therefore older couples may develop sexual difficulties independently of

A. Gregory (✉)
Department of Sexual Health, Chandos Clinic, Nottingham University Hospital Trust, Nottingham, UK
e-mail: Angela.Gregory@nuh.nhs.uk

© Springer Nature Switzerland AG 2021
A. Rantell (ed.), *Sexual Function and Pelvic Floor Dysfunction*,
https://doi.org/10.1007/978-3-030-63843-6_15

each other and it is important to enquire about a partner's sexual health and establish how satisfactory their sexual relationship was prior to the onset of their own or their partner's particular difficulties. The onset of sexual problems in one partner can also result in emotional or sexual issues for the other especially when avoidance is a major factor. Feelings of loss, resentment, rejection and emotional distress are common. This creates challenges in relationships by causing further distress which supports and maintains sexual difficulties. Men or women not in a sexual partnership face further challenges around performance anxiety in the context of a new relationship and it can be helpful to listen to their concerns and discuss communication strategies. For example, women concerned about painful penetration could use vaginal trainers (dilators) discussed in Chap. 12, to improve confidence and reduce anxiety about pain. Men, concerned about ED could be encouraged to take things slowly with a new sexual partner and not pressure themselves into feeling that they 'should' have penetration as soon as their relationship becomes intimate. This reduces anxiety, promotes arousal and improves confidence irrespective of whether they are using ED medication or not. Clinical experience indicates that communicating about sexual concerns often proves difficult even for those in established relationships and rehearsing options of what to say and when to say it can be helpful. It is advisable to discuss avoidance of intimacy or sexual concerns outside of the bedroom. Some prefer to write their partner a letter or find it easier to talk outside of the home by going for a drive or a walk; it's often easier to discuss difficult subjects when not looking directly at one another.

15.2 Erectile Dysfunction

When assessing *all* sexual difficulties, it is essential to enquire whether the problem is primary (lifelong) or secondary (acquired), generalised or situational.

Definition: '*the inability to obtain and maintain an erection or decreased erectile rigidity despite adequate sexual stimulation. This must occur 75%–100% of the time for a period of at least six months duration*' (American Psychiatric Association 2013).

The pioneering research by Masters and Johnson in the 1960s concluded that all sexual difficulties were psychological or relational in origin. However, the medical research stimulated by the launch of Viagra (Sildenafil) on the 27th March 1998, the first oral therapy for erectile dysfunction followed in 2003, by Cialis (Tadalafil) and Levitra (Vardenafil), challenged this well-established belief. For the first time there was undeniable evidence of the impact of organic causes such as diabetes, cardiovascular disease, spinal cord injury, prostate surgery, hypogonadism, thyroid disease, multiple sclerosis and Parkinson's disease on erectile function (Porst 2012a). Men should seek treatment at the earliest opportunity to ensure that any underlying health condition is addressed. Psychogenic causes of ED are performance anxiety, loss of sexual self-confidence inexperience, relationship distress and partner sexual difficulties. Anxiety about performance triggers adrenalin and noradrenalin, elevates the sympathetic nervous system and constricts the penile smooth muscle, the primary cause of psychogenic ED; it can also be significant in men with organic ED (Kirana and Porst 2012).

15.2.1 Medical History

Often sexual dysfunction is multi-factorial therefore it is necessary to identify all *maintaining* factors including organic causes and prescribed medications. ED and cardio vascular disease (CVD) frequently coexist and ED may be an early warning sign for occult CVD with window of opportunity for CVD risk reduction of 2–5 years (Jackson et al. 2010). There is evidence that regular physical activity and weight loss can significantly improve erectile function, efficacy of Phosphodiesterase-5 inhibitors (PDE5i's) and reduce the risk of cardiovascular diseases/events with benefits being seen as early as 8 weeks after initiation (Jackson et al. 2010).

Education helps patients understand how the body works, normalises their experiences, especially around age/disease related changes and highlights possible reasons for unsuccessful pharmacological treatment. It also provides an opportunity to explain the role of performance anxiety, common in both organic and psychogenic erectile dysfunction. Performance anxiety is the fear of future sexual failure based on previous failures it interferes with sexual arousal, distracts from sensual feelings, undermines sexual self-confidence and ultimately contributes to sexual avoidance (Tripodi et al. 2012).

First-line treatment for erectile dysfunction is Phosphodiesterase-5 inhibitors (PDE5i) for those men for whom this is contraindicated; other options include intracavernosal injections, vacuum devices, urethral alprostadil and finally penile prosthesis. The British Society of Sexual Medicine (BSSM) provides an assessment algorism and treatment guidelines (Hackett et al. 2018). Assessment should include questions about any previous treatments psychological or pharmacological. If PDE5 inhibitors have been prescribed, then detailed questions should be asked about which medications were tried, at what dose, how many were taken, the context in which they were used and what response was achieved. The answers will highlight what needs to be addressed to optimise future success. A lack of education, inadequate dosing, insufficient medication, negative side effects, unrealistic expectations, performance anxiety or partner's response are some of the many for reasons for failure. Several sponsored and non-sponsored studies have investigated whether patient/couples prefer one drug over another once they have been offered the opportunity to try them all over a reasonably long period. A recent literature review (2000–2010) of patients' preference studies concluded 52–65% preferred tadalafil compared to vardenafil 12–20% and sildenafil 8–30%. The reasons for the preference were mainly due to the longer duration of action and increased spontaneity (Porst 2012a). Spontaneity reduces performance anxiety as the patient can take a tablet well ahead of any hoped for, expected or planned sexual activity. Therefore it is essential that patient preference should be taken into consideration.

15.3   Ejaculatory Dysfunction

After ED the most common male sexual dysfunction is premature ejaculation (Porst 2012b). A number of medical and therapeutic interventions exist; however, there is no first-line treatment for premature ejaculation and men should be assessed and treated on a case by case basis. Most cases seen in clinical practice are related to inexperience, masturbatory habit, inability to control arousal, performance anxiety and relationship distress.

15.3.1 Premature Ejaculation

Definition: '*A persistent or recurrent pattern of ejaculation occurring during part-nered sexual activity within approximately 1 minutes following penetration and before the person wishes it, this must occur 75%–100% of the time for a period of at least six months duration*' (American Psychiatric Association 2013).

A number of selective serotonin reuptake inhibitors are currently used off-label in long-term daily dosing regimens to treat PE (McCarty and Dinsmore 2012). The results are variable with some experiencing significant improvement but others with little or no improvement. Unpleasant side effects can also make continuation difficult. In 2013, dapoxetine (Priligy), an SSRI with a short half-life received a treatment licence for the treatment of PE. A mixture of prilocaine and lidocaine has also been shown to improve ejaculatory latency and control (Dinsmore and Wyllie 2009). There is a general consensus that the psychosexual therapy offers additional benefits for patients with PE (Althof 2013). This may include a masturbatory re-training programme, relaxation techniques, pelvic floor relaxation and breathing techniques and couple strategies including sensate focus. Medical Note—Primary (lifelong) PE findings support a genetic component and hyperthyroidism is a hormonal risk factor for acquired PE with incidence rates of between 50 and 60% (Porst 2012b).

15.3.2 Delayed Ejaculation

Definition: '*A persistent difficulty or inability to achieve ejaculation despite the presence of adequate desire, arousal and stimulation*' that the clinician, taking into account the person's age, judges to be adequate in focus, intensity and duration'. *The disturbance causes marked distress or interpersonal difficulties and must occur 75%–100% of the time for a period of at least six months duration* (American Psychiatric Association 2013).

Men with primary inhibited ejaculation in all situations should be investigated to exclude any physical causes, e.g. those who find it difficult to retract their foreskin during masturbation/penetration require a clinical evaluation. However, the most common presentation are men who can orgasm and ejaculate during masturbation but not during partner sex. In such cases, masturbatory frequency, pornography use or an idiosyncratic masturbatory style are often significant *maintaining* factors. If an idiosyncratic masturbatory style is identified, then a masturbatory re-training programme can be initiated which incorporates a position and stimulation that more closely reflects penetration. Re-training takes time and needs to be carried out regularly to challenge the well-established conditioning nature of the previous stimulus. Some men get into the habit of 'trying hard' to ejaculate during penetration which negatively impacts on both relaxation and arousal and establishes a pattern of performance anxiety with similar inhibitory effects to those experienced by men with ED. Clear boundaries about stopping penetration before it becomes 'hard work' or uncomfortable should be discussed and advice about using manual stimulation to achieve ejaculation could be suggested. Medical Note—Diabetes, prostate surgery, spinal cord injury, MS and some medications can also impact on a man's ability to ejaculate. Anejaculation describes a complete lack of ejaculate due to retrograde ejaculation when the semen overcomes the internal sphincter barrier and empties into the bladder (Porst and Cruz 2012). Men who have undergone a radical prostatectomy are unable to ejaculate due to the removal of the prostate but their ability to orgasm remains intact.

15.4   Male Hypoactive Sexual Desire Disorder

Definition: '*persistently or recurrently deficient (or absent) sexual/erotic thoughts or fantasies and desire for sexual activity*', *as judged by a clinician with consideration for the patient's age and cultural context* (American Psychiatric Association 2013).

Typically men are only diagnosed with one of three subtypes of HSD:

- Primary/generalised: The man has little or no desire for sexual stimulation (with a partner or alone) and never had.
- Secondary/generalised: The man previously had sexual interest in his present partner, but lacks interest in sexual activity, partnered or solitary.
- Secondary/situational: The man was previously sexually interested in his present partner but now lacks sexual interest in this partner but has desire for sexual stimulation (i.e. alone or with someone other than his present partner).

It has also been found that decreased partner's libido and partner illness significantly contribute to a lack of sexual desire and that the presence of menopausal symptoms can lead to low sexual desire in her partner. In addition, a long relationship span could reduce partner's sex appeal and the patient's desire (Corona et al. 2013a).

Medical Note—As with women, various medical problems, partner sexual problems, psychiatric problems (such as mood disorders), medication, pain, relationship distress, general stress and anxiety can impact on male sexual interest. Also increased amounts of prolactin or low levels of testosterone can result in HSD (Corona et al. 2013b).

15.4.1 Masturbation

15.4.1.1 Physical and Psychological Benefits

Whilst there is little in terms of validated evidence regarding the health benefits of masturbation, we do know that sexual arousal either partner or solo stimulated increases blood flow which improves the endothelial function of erectile tissue in both men and women. During arousal dopamine is released along with other neurotransmitters such as serotonin, endorphins and oxytocin which can improve mood and induce feelings of relaxation as well as offering pain relief. Masturbation is a way for those not in a relationship or those in relationships were there are differences in sexual interest to meet their own personal sexual needs. For single women who have never masturbated or who feel uncomfortable or inhibited doing so explaining these benefits can be helpful. If a women hopes to meet a sexual partner in the future she should be encouraged to explore and accept her body especially after age or disease-related changes. Discussing the use of sex toys in a clinical context gives the subject validity and provides 'permission' for a women to consider this as an option. If a woman is or was in a same sex relationship, it is important to clarify whether penetration is an important aspect for them. If the answer is yes, then the benefits of maintaining comfortable penetration should be encouraged especially for those with symptoms related to the menopause such as vaginal dryness or atrophy, incontinence or prolapse. If not, alternatives such as outercourse, regular clitoral stimulation or clitoral vacuum devices alongside the benefits of using a vaginal moisturiser could be suggested. Orgasm alone or with a partner involves the pelvic floor so advice regarding maintaining a healthy pelvic floor for both men and women is important. **Medical Note**—Women (or men) with pelvic floor hypertonicity should be encouraged to relax and stretch the muscles of the pelvic floor.

Research suggests that many people masturbate yet its role is often neglected by researchers and health care professional's alike (Laumann et al. 1994; Johnson et al. 1990). The Natsal Survey questioned men about whether they had masturbated in the previous 4 weeks and found that the mean average was 66.4% over all age groups between 16 and 74 years (Mercer et al. 2013). It also found that twice as many men than women reported masturbating in the previous 4 weeks with proportions decreasing steadily with age in men but falling only after the age of 55 years in women (Mercer et al. 2013). The incidence of sexual intercourse also decreased in this age group which is of concern given that women aged 55 years and over are most at risk of vaginal dryness, vaginal atrophy, lack of lubrication, reduced sexual interest/arousal and orgasmic capacity.

15.4.1.2 Male Masturbation

Of all the sexual practices it remains one that few enquire about or discuss (Lipsith et al. 2003). Over 20 years ago Perelman reported that in his clinical experience masturbatory frequency and technique were often implicated in difficulties with male sexual desire, erection and ejaculation and that specific details about masturbation provide a wealth of diagnostic information (Perelman 1994).

Erectile Dysfunction—Questions about masturbation can identify whether a man's ED is situational and help diagnose whether his ED is primarily psychogenic in nature. Accessibility to online hard core pornography can result in high frequency viewing and masturbation which can have a conditioning effect and negatively impact on a man's ability to become aroused during partnered sex. It is also common for men with ED to masturbate in an attempt to 'test out' their erectile responses, paying little attention to feelings of sexual desire or arousal often leading to further failure. Alternatively men who are struggling with their erectile responses due to organic factors may be encouraged to masturbate especially if they are not in a sexual relationship or if penetration occurs infrequently the aim is to help restore confidence (alongside medical treatment) and improve the endothelial function of the penile tissue.

Premature Ejaculation—Asking about masturbatory technique can help identify if a man has learnt any control of his arousal during self-stimulation. Questions about speed of stimulation, privacy and pornography use can help identify factors potentially creating heightened physiological and psychological responses which could 'trigger' rapid ejaculation thereby highlighting whether a masturbatory retraining programme would be beneficial. For men with PE this includes varying physiological and psychological stimulation using a variety of techniques and is useful for men that have not learnt how to control their sexual arousal during self-stimulation. Once learnt, such techniques can then be applied to controlling arousal during penetration (Metz and McCarthy 2003).

Delayed Ejaculation—If this only occurs during partnered sex, it is essential to ask about masturbation frequency and pornography use. Highly arousing material and/or vigorous stimulation can result in a man finding it difficult to achieve similar arousal/stimulation during partnered sex. Asking about masturbatory technique can also identify an idiosyncratic style that includes very specific stimulation or a physical position unlikely to be experienced during penetration, thus making it difficult to achieve sufficient levels of sexual arousal to facilitate orgasm and ejaculation. Such detail can provide valuable information for inclusion into a masturbatory retraining programme.

Hypoactive sexual desire—Questions about masturbation are helpful in assessing whether the problem is generalised or situational. For example, a man who regularly masturbates but is not interested in partner sex indicates that the issue may be partner related perhaps as a result of relationship distress or that their partner experiences sexual function issues. Questions related to whether there are concerns about erectile function with a partner can highlight whether their problem is secondary to worries related to erectile dysfunction as opposed to that of low sexual desire.

15.4.1.3   Female Masturbation

Orgasmic Disorder—For women who present with absent or diminished orgasmic responses self-pleasuring exercises or therapeutic masturbation can be introduced. Self-pleasuring/masturbation involves a series of skills beginning with body awareness/acceptance, non-genital body exploration, genital exploration, erotic stimulation, using erotic fantasies, multiple stimulation including vibrators and/or clitoral suction devices, using 'orgasm triggers' such as pulsing the pelvic floor muscles or tensing both legs together (Metz et al. 2018).

Sexual/genital pain—A lack of arousal can be the 'trigger' for initial sexual discomfort or be the result of previous negative pain experiences. Specific suggestions to improve arousal give a woman permission to explore what she finds sexually stimulating and is helpful especially when used in conjunction with vaginal trainers (dilators). This may include clear boundaries for a couple not to attempt penetration but to focus on massage and sensual touch and teasing.

Sexual Interest/arousal disorder—Physiological and psychological relaxation is essential to experience improved sensation and levels of arousal. The benefits of mindfulness in sexuality have been increasingly recognised in recent years, with a growing number of clinicians integrating the practice of non-judgemental attention into the moment to moment experience as an important part of the sexual treatment (Carvalheira and Vilarinho 2013). Mindfulness has been used effectively as part of a group treatment programme for women with sexual complaints secondary to gynaecological cancer. The programme was specifically developed to target sexual arousal complaints in women after a radical hysterectomy due to cervical or endometrial cancer (Brotto and Heiman 2007).

15.4.1.4   The Impact of Male Sexual Difficulties

Female partners of men with ED frequently report a decrease in sexual interest and levels of arousal, as well as reduced frequency of orgasm and satisfaction with sexual activity following the onset of their partner's erectile difficulties (Corona and Maggi 2013). On the other hand, a non-intimate and non-loving relationship or sexual interest and/or performance problems in the female partner could exacerbate male sexual dysfunction. The rejected partner feels hurt and confused and may withdraw emotionally or become angry and resentful so that the difficulty is compounded further by relationship disharmony.

It has also been reported that PE can lead to inadequate central and genital arousal, vaginal dryness and inability to orgasm in their female partner (Graziottin and Althof 2011). A survey of more than 1400 partners of men suffering from PE showed that the inappropriate attention focus of the man and his avoidance of other forms of sexual activities represented the main source of women's sexual distress (Burri et al. 2014).

The recognition of the negative impact of male sexual dysfunction on their partner's sexual life means that treatment centred on the couple rather than individual is often more successful. For example in clinical practice men are regularly referred for psychosexual therapy when medication alone has not proved successful in the treatment of their erectile dysfunction, regardless of aetiology. Whilst there may be medical reasons for this often it's related to avoidance, lack of communication, relationship distress, how their partner has responded to the issue or finally sexual concerns of their own. Addressing these during therapy can maximise the effectiveness of medical intervention. However, most studies identify women's integration into therapy only as an effective strategy in the management of the male's sexual problems. Given the negative impact of common sexual/genital complaints particularly around the time of the menopause it is evident from clinical practice that such complaints impact both on the women herself and her male partner. This may be related to avoidance of intimate and sexual contact resulting in feelings of rejection and also directly on male sexual function. It can be difficult to perform and maintain an erection especially if a man feels that his partner is unresponsive to his advances, visibly tensing or experiences pain prior to or during penetration. In a small study of 17 heterosexual couples seeking sex therapy for vaginismus found that erectile dysfunction was the most frequently reported male sexual difficulty (Klein et al. 2015).

15.4.1.5   The Impact of Female Sexual Difficulties

Common sexual complaints at menopause, such as vaginal dryness and painful sex, lack of sexual interest/arousal and poor sexual satisfaction, should be routinely assessed in clinical practice in order to preserve quality of life across the ageing process, especially in surgically or medically induced menopausal women in whom sexual symptoms may be more distressing (Caruso and Malandrino 2013). In fact expert opinion recommends non-hormonal vaginal lubricants and moisturisers, as well as ongoing sexual activity, as a first-line treatment for symptomatic vaginal dryness and atrophy (North American Menopause Society (NAMS) 2007). Regular intercourse provides protection from atrophy by increasing the blood flow to the pelvic organs (Lev-Sagie and Nyirjesy 2009). However from a practical point of view painful intercourse is difficult to sustain therefore it is essential that women are encouraged and educated on the benefits of these preparations. For women without a partner or those who have experienced long periods of sexual abstinence, the use of vaginal trainers (dilators) or a vibrator can help restore sexual self-confidence, manage anticipatory anxiety related to pain/penetration and maintain the vaginal integrity when used alongside a lubricant and moisturiser.

One study that investigated the impact of provoked vulvodynia (PVD) on the couple found that partners of women who experience dyspareunia secondary to PVD report a primarily negative impact of that pain on their own psychological and sexual health (Sadownik et al. 2017). Clinicians in this field should explicitly inquire not only about the couple's relationship health, but also about the male partner's psychological and sexual health. To date, PVD has largely been framed as a woman's problem, and the treatments, and treatment outcomes, have predominantly focused only on the women themselves. This study suggests that for some men it is important to find a place where partners can express their experiences coping with PVD whilst connecting with other partners with similar experiences. Finally, support systems may be desirable for partners—for example, online groups, in-person informal meetings or facilitated formal meetings. This study is one of the first qualitative studies to involve partners of women with PVD and adds to a growing literature highlighting the impact of PVD on partners and the importance of including them in treatment.

The integrity of the supportive structures of the lower genital tract is not given its due consideration as causative factors for sexual pain (Davis and Brooks 2009). Pelvic organ prolapse (POP) can be a significant cause of vaginal and rectal pressure and pain. In addition, women with POP frequently complain that they have a sensation of 'bulging' or that 'something is falling out'. POP can also cause incontinence of urine or stool. Because of these factors POP presents significant barriers to sexual function. In addition POP may exacerbate other vulvar diseases that may in themselves cause sexual dysfunction. For example, urinary incontinence (UI) may worsen the symptoms of lichen sclerosis (Davis and Brooks 2009). Urinary incontinence occurs in up to 25% of older women during intercourse. This condition commonly leads to dissatisfaction with their sexual relationship or more frequently to withdrawal from sexual contact because of embarrassment. Urinary tract symptoms can be predictors of lubrication insufficiency, orgasmic dysfunction and dyspareunia (Corona and Maggi 2013).

Whilst several studies have identified the impact of UI on women's sexual functioning and satisfaction, the effects of UI on the functioning of their male partners was unknown (Bekker et al. 2010). However in one study women attending an outpatient appointment for urological assessment and their partners were asked to complete the Golombok Rust Inventory of Sexual Satisfaction questionnaire (GRISS). Of the 189 couples who completed the questionnaires 42.9% of the women reported UI. The women with UI demonstrated lower overall SF, lower frequency of intercourse, were more likely to show avoidance behaviour and have more problems with communication. Men with partners with UI also reported an overall diminished SF, lower frequency of intercourse, reduced satisfaction and were more likely to have erectile problems. However, there were no questions as to whose problems started first (Bekker et al. 2010).

A further study using face to face interviews with 32 incontinent women who reported urinary leakage during intercourse and 60 asymptomatic controls, found that incontinent women were 4.7 times less satisfied with their sexual lives when compared to the control group and their partners had ejaculation without full erection 3.1 more times (which may have added to the decreased satisfaction). During these interviews several methods of coping with leakage during intercourse were volunteered and these are shown in Table 15.1 below (Beji et al. 2005).

Table 15.1 Methods of coping adopted by women with leakage problems during intercourse

Ways of coping with problems	N	%
Micturating prior to sexual intercourse	6	18.8
Keeping the partner unaware of the problem	16	50
Deferring intercourse	9	28.1
Partner suggests anal coitus	2	6.3
Ignoring the problem	8	25
Interrupting intercourse prematurely	6	18.8

Again another study that focused on a carer's perspective of the effect of incontinence on sexuality found that although UI did not affect sexual intimacy, it did affect sexual intercourse and sleeping in separate bedrooms was common. Faecal incontinence was found to have a far greater effect on SF than UI (Cassells and Watt 2003).

15.5 Conclusion

Partnership conflict, relationship imbalance, commitment issues, intimacy and communication problems, lack of trust, mismatches in sexual desire, boredom and poor sexual techniques are just some of the common sources of sexual dissatisfaction noted among couples of all ages (Corona and Maggi 2013). Sexual problems are sometimes the cause and sometimes the result of dysfunctional or unsatisfactory relationships. It is often difficult to determine which came first as the research literature is conflicting (Silvaggi and Tripodi 2013). However, several studies consistently demonstrate the interdependence of sexual function between partners. Specifically they suggest that dysfunction in one partner tends to cause problems for the other and improvement in function tends to have a positive effect on their partner. The preponderance of evidence suggests that therapy which specifically addresses couple issues will be more successful than therapy or treatment that only focuses on the resolution of sexual dysfunction (Silvaggi and Tripodi 2013). Finally the evidence suggests that Masters and Johnson 1966 were accurate when they stated 'that there is no such thing as an uninvolved partner in a relationship where sexual dysfunction exists'.

As a clinician caring for a woman reporting sexual dysfunction it is essential to consider that their SDF may not solely be due to their own physical or psychological problems, but may be significantly impacted by issues/health concerns experienced by the partner.

References

Althof S (2013) Integrated and combined therapy. In: Kirana PS, Tripoldi F, Reisman Y, Porst H (eds) The EFS & ESSM syllabus of clinical sexology. Medix, Amsterdam

American Psychiatric Association (2013) Diagnostic and statistical manual of mental disorders, 5th edn. American Psychiatric Press, Washington, DC

Beji NK, Yalcın O, Ayyildiz EH, Kayir A (2005) Effect of urinary leakage on sexual function during sexual intercourse. Urol Int 74(3):250–255

Bekker MD, Beck JJ, Putter H, Van Driel MF, Pelger R, Weijmar Schultz WC, Lycklama à Nijeholt GA, Elzevier HW (2010) Sexual experiences of men with incontinent partners. J Sex Med 7(5):1877–1882

Brotto LA, Heiman JR (2007) Mindfulness in sex therapy: applications for women with sexual difficulties following gynecologic cancer. Sex Relat Ther 22(1):3–11

Burri A, Giuliano F, McMahon C, Porst H (2014) Female partner's perception of premature ejaculation and its impact on relationship break-up, relationship quality and sexual satisfaction. J Sex Med 11:2243–2255

Caruso S, Malandrino C (2013) Menopause and female sexuality. In: Kirana PS, Tripoldi F, Reisman Y, Porst H (eds) The EFS & ESSM syllabus of clinical sexology. Medix, Amsterdam

Carvalheira AA, Vilarinho S (2013) Mindfulness for sexual problems. In: Kirana PS, Tripoldi F, Reisman Y, Porst H (eds) The EFS & ESSM syllabus of clinical sexology. Medix, Amsterdam

Cassells C, Watt E (2003) The impact of incontinence on older spousal caregivers. J Adv Nurs 42(6):607–616

Corona G, Maggi M (2013) Sexuality in the elderly population. In: Reisman Y, Porst H (eds) The ESSM syllabus of sexual medicine. Medix, Amsterdam

Corona G, Rastrelli G, Ricca V, Jannini EA, Vignozzi L, Monami M et al (2013a) Risks factors with primary and secondary reduced libido in male patients sexual dysfunction. J Sex Med 10:1074–1089

Corona G et al (2013b) Male hypoactive sexual desire disorder. In: Kirana PS, Tripoldi F, Reisman Y, Porst H (eds) The EFS & ESSM syllabus of clinical sexology. Medix, Amsterdam

Damsted PC (2012) Female sexual function in midlife. In: Reisman Y, Porst H (eds) The ESSM syllabus of sexual medicine. Medix, Amsterdam

Davis G, Brooks J (2009) Pelvic organ prolapse and sexual pain. In: Goldstein A, Pukhall C, Goldstein I (eds) Female sexual pain disorders. Wiley Blackwell, Chichester

Dinsmore WW, Wyllie MG (2009) PSD502 improves ejaculatory latency, control and sexual satisfaction when applied topically 5 mins before intercourse in men with premature ejaculation: results of a phase 11, multicentre, double blind, placebo-controlled study. BJU Int 103:940–949

Graziottin A, Althof S (2011) What does premature ejaculation mean to the man, the woman, and the couple? J Sex Med 8:S304–S309

Hackett G, Kirby M, Wylie K, Heald A, Ossei-Gerning N, Edwards D, Muneer A (2018) British Society for Sexual Medicine Guidelines on the management of erectile dysfunction in men. J Sex Med 15:430–457

Jackson G et al (2010) Erectile dysfunction and coronary artery disease prediction: evidence based guidance and consensus. Int J Clin Pract 64(7):848–857

Johnson AM et al (1990) The national survey of sexual attitudes and lifestyles. S.C.P.R, London

Kirana E, Porst H (2012) Erectile dysfunction. In: Kirana E, Tripoldi Fm Reisman Y, Porst H (eds) The EFS & ESSM syllabus of sexual medicine. Medix, Amsterdam

Klein V et al (2015) Sexual history of male partners of women with the diagnosis vaginismus. Sex Relat Ther 30:376–384

Laumann EO et al (1994) The social organisation of sexuality. University of Chicago Press, Chicago

Lev-Sagie A, Nyirjesy P (2009) Noninfectious vaginitis. In: Goldstein A, Pukhall C, Goldstein I (eds) Female sexual pain disorders. Wiley Blackwell, Chichester

Lipsith J, McCann D, Goldmeier D (2003) Male psychogenic sexual dysfunction: the role of masturbation. J Sex Relat Ther 18(4):447–471

Masters WH, Johnson VE (1966) Human sexual response. Churchill, London

McCarty EJ, Dinsmore WW (2012) Dapoxetine: an evidence-based review of its effectiveness in treatment of premature ejaculation. Dove Medical Press, London

Mercer CH et al (2013) Changes in sexual attitudes and lifestyles in Britain through the life course and over time: findings from the National Surveys of sexual attitudes and lifestyles (Natsal). Lancet 382:1781–1794

Metz E, McCarthy W (2003) Coping with premature ejaculation. New Harbinger, Oakland, CA

Metz E, Epstein NB, McCarthy W (2018) Cognitive—behavioural therapy for sexual dysfunction. Routledge, New York

North American Menopause Society (NAMS) (2007) The role of local vaginal estrogen for treatment of vaginal atrophy in postmenopausal women. Position statement of NAMS. Menopause 14:357–369

Perelman MA (1994) Masturbation revisited. Contemp Urol 6:67–80

Porst H (2012a) Erectile dysfunction. In: Reisman Y, Porst H (eds) The ESSM syllabus of sexual medicine. Medix, Amsterdam

Porst H (2012b) Premature Ejaculation. In: Reisman Y, Porst H (eds) The ESSM syllabus of sexual medicine. Medix, Amsterdam

Porst H, Cruz N (2012) Basic Anatomy and physiology of ejaculation, classification of ejacula-
    tory disorders. In: Reisman Y, Porst H (eds) The ESSM syllabus of sexual medicine. Medix,
    Amsterdam
Sadownik A, Smith KB, Brotto LA (2017) The impact of a woman's dyspareunia and its treatment
    on her intimate partner: a qualitative analysis. J Sex Marital Ther 43(6):529–542
Silvaggi C, Tripodi F (2013) Psychological barriers to sexual functioning. In: Kirana PS, Tripoldi
    F, Reisman Y, Porst H (eds) The EFS & ESSM syllabus of clinical sexology. Medix, Amsterdam
Tripodi F, Silvagg C, Simonelli C (2012) Psychology of sexual response. In: Porst H, Reisman Y
    (eds) The ESSM syllabus of sexual medicine. Medix, Amsterdam

.

Access to Services and Help-Seeking Behaviour

16

Angie Rantell

16.1 Introduction

Health or care seeking behaviour has been defined as any action undertaken by individuals who perceive themselves to have a health problem or to be ill for the purpose of finding an appropriate remedy (Editorial Health Seeking Behaviour in Context 2003). In general, help-seeking behaviours are dependent upon three categories, attitudes (beliefs and willingness) towards help seeking, intention to seek help, and actual help-seeking behaviour (Gulliver et al. 2012).

The prevalence of help seeking for individuals describing sexual problems has been reported between 10% and 21% (Štulhofer et al. 2020; Moreira et al. 2005; Mercer et al. 2003). Whereas, help seeking for women with pelvic floor dysfunction (PFD) has been reported between 20 and 83.1% (Seim et al. 1995, McDowell et al. 1996; Tinetti et al. 2018). There are potentially many reasons for this including the level of bothersomeness of symptoms and impact on everyday quality of life. In many cases, help seeking may be dependent on the primary complaint and for many women, this would generally be the PFD. However, it does not mean that the SDF should not be addressed at the same time.

16.2 Factors Associated with Help Seeking

In the literature, there are several factors associated with help seeking. In a study of women with PFD, increased symptom bother was the main factor associated with help seeking (Tinetti et al. 2018). Whereas in the study considering the extent of SF in the general population in the UK, people with persistent problems were more likely to have sought help (Mercer et al. 2003).

A. Rantell (✉)
Urogynaecology Department, King's College Hospital, London, UK
e-mail: angela.rantell@nhs.net

In a population based survey conducted on sexual difficulties and associated sexual distress in Belgium, 43.5% of women reported a moderate to severe sexual difficulty. Sexual distress was associated with more sexual dissatisfaction and greater sexual avoidance. Sexual distress also was associated with help-seeking behaviour (Hendrickx et al. 2016).

16.3   Factors That Hinder Help Seeking

It has been reported that patients do not always communicate their concerns to their health care professional (HCP), through either embarrassment or misconceptions of what is a 'medical problem' (Shaw et al. 2001). This is further compounded by the stereotypical perception that HCPs do not understand the relevance of SF. The possibility of the HCP's dismissive reaction and lack of understanding has also been reported to impact upon help seeking (Schaller et al. 2020; Gott and Hinchliff 2003; Hinchliff and Gott 2011).

The concept of embarrassment in health care has been proven to deter patients from seeking help (McKie 1993), add to the discomfort of chronic problems such as UI (United States Department of Health and Human Services Publications 1992), and deter staff from broaching the topic of sexual function (Kelleher and Oxenham 1993). However, it is not just the embarrassment of the patient that is a barrier but also that of the clinician. Meerabeau (1999) performed a review of the literature on embarrassment, in healthcare, particularly related to consultations/examinations related to sexual issues. She summarised that 'the current literature indicates that nurses and doctors have not shed the understandings acquired in their primary socialisation, which has taught us that sexuality is a private affair'. It could be considered that helping HCPs to overcome their embarrassment should be the first point of training, before trying to break down the patient barriers to facilitate effective communication on issues of SF.

Personal discomfort and embarrassment regarding SA has been established as a barrier to help-seeking behaviour in women (Nicolosi et al. 2006) and symptoms of PFD e.g. urgency incontinence are especially associated with feelings of embarrassment (Brown et al. 1998; Van der Vaart et al. 2002; Norton 2003).

Other reasons for not seeking help for SDF reported in a study by Vahdaninia (2009) include (Vahdaninia et al. 2009):

- Doctor cannot help me.
- I had time constraints.
- It did not occur to me.
- I was not asked about my problems.
- The problem is a normal part of getting older.

It has been suggested that help seeking reflects an awareness of the availability of treatments and advice for these disorders (Mercer et al. 2003) and therefor by improving public health and awareness of SDF it may encourage help seeking.

Improving the HCP's communication skills and ensuring that the broach the topic would again resolve some of these barriers identified.

Many women adopt coping mechanisms to manage their sexual problems and the most common coping mechanism reported by up to 64.3% of women is avoidance of sexual activity (Mercer et al. 2003). Therefore, when broaching the topic of SA, when a woman reports that she is not sexually active, it is essential to understand why, to ensure that problems are not missed.

16.4   Access to Services

There are significant variations regarding access to therapies around the world. This is due to the various different health systems in place. In those countries without a National Health Service, there may be significant inequalities in access to services due to costs of services and limitations in what personal insurance will cover. In countries where health services are readily available, free/affordable access to services may be limited by geographical constraints as specialist sexual services are not always available in all locations or by a lack of specialist services.

For many women, when they first recognise/accept that they have an issue, the internet is often the first place that they would look to for advice or information. Although there are many reputable sources that provide high quality information, there is also a lot of information provided from less reliable sources and for patients it can be difficult to know what advice to follow.

The International Society for the Study of Women's Sexual Health (ISSWSH) is a multidisciplinary, academic, and scientific organisation that provides support and education for HCPs and researchers working in the field of women's sexual health. The society also focus on providing the public with accurate information about women's sexuality and sexual health. As such, their website lists many different education resources for HCPs and patients as well as links to other reputable sources of information.

Most women seeking help for SDF would generally present to their General Practitioner (GP) or family doctor (Štulhofer et al. 2020). It would usually be expected that they perform an initial assessment to determine the most appropriate service to further investigate/manage the woman's concern, e.g. gynaecologist/sexual therapist and they would then make the necessary referral. Most commonly, a multi-disciplinary team approach is necessary and joint working between services and practitioners should be encouraged. Having a knowledge of specialist services and practitioners in the local area and their specific referral criteria pathways is essential knowledge when caring for women with PFD.

Some women, however, may not want to discuss issues regarding SF with a family doctor and may wish to seek help directly and see a specialist privately. Yet, how are women to know which services will provide the highest standards of care? The ISSWSH website does offer a 'Find a provider' tool that allows women to type in their location and will advise them regarding registered local practitioners. Although this is an International database, only ISSWSH members are listed so women may also consider a more local recommendation. Many countries will have a National Professional body that providers will be accredited with. For example in the UK, sexual therapists can register to be an accredited member of the College of Sexual and Relationship Therapists (COSRT). This means they will be fully qualified and able to advise on physical, psychological, and medical factors that can affect sexual well-being. The COSRT Register contains details of qualified, specialist psychosexual and/or relationship therapists. These members have demonstrated high professional standards and meet strict training, experience and benchmarks. Signposting women to these resources can help them to access safe and accredited services.

16.5 Conclusions

Although the number of women seeking help for SDF is low, this does not mean that women do not want help. HCP should be actively involved in the holistic care of women and this includes sexual health. Therefore, a fundamental role of the HCP is in introducing the topic of SF to women and asking if they experience any sexual issues. Once these have been identified, women can be directed to or advised on how to access appropriate services. For those who do not wish to access services directly, HCPs can still provide advice on free sources of information/help that women can access on line.

References

Brown JS, Subak LL, GRAS J, Brown BA, Kuppermann M, Posner SF (1998) Urge incontinence: the patient's perspective. J Womens Health 7(10):1263–1269

Editorial Health Seeking Behaviour in Context (2003). Available from http://www.ajol.info/index. php/eamj/article/viewFile/8689/1927

Gott M, Hinchliff S (2003) Barriers to seeking treatment for sexual problems in primary care: a qualitative study with older people. Fam Pract 20(6):690–695

Gulliver A, Griffiths KM, Christensen H, Brewer JL (2012) A systematic review of help-seeking interventions for depression, anxiety and general psychological distress. BMC Psychiatry 12(1):81

Hendrickx L, Gijs L, Enzlin P (2016) Sexual difficulties and associated sexual distress in Flanders (Belgium): a representative population-based survey study. J Sex Med 13(4):650–668

Hinchliff S, Gott M (2011) Seeking medical help for sexual concerns in mid-and later life: a review of the literature. J Sex Res 48(2–3):106–117

Kelleher A, Oxenham J (1993) An open approach to a delicate subject. Management of diabetes related sexual problems. Prof Nurse 8(7):465–468

McDowell BJ, Engberg SJ, Rodriguez E, Engberg R, Sereika S (1996) Characteristics of urinary incontinence in homebound older adults. J Am Geriatr Soc 44:963–968

McKie L (1993) Women's views of the cervical smear test: implications for nursing practice. J Adv Nurs 18(8):1228–1234

Meerabeau L (1999) The management of embarrassment and sexuality in health care. J Adv Nurs 29(6):1507–1513

Mercer CH, Fenton KA, Johnson AM, Wellings K, Macdowall W, McManus S, Nanchahal K, Erens B (2003) Sexual function problems and help seeking behaviour in Britain: national probability sample survey. BMJ 327(7412):426–427

Moreira ED, Glasser DB, Gingell C (2005) Sexual activity, sexual dysfunction and associated help-seeking behaviours in middle-aged and older adults in Spain: a population survey. World J Urol 23(6):422–429

Nicolosi A, Buvat J, Glasser DB, Hartmann U, Laumann EO, Gingell C (2006) Sexual behaviour, sexual dysfunctions and related help seeking patterns in middle-aged and elderly Europeans: the global study of sexual attitudes and behaviors. World J Urol 24(4):423–428

Norton C (2003) OAB evidence from the patient's perspective. Eur Urol Suppl 2(5):16–22

Schaller S, Traeen B, Lundin Kvalem I (2020) Barriers and facilitating factors in help-seeking: a qualitative study on how older adults experience talking about sexual issues with healthcare personnel. Int J Sex Health 32:65–80

Seim A, Sandvik H, Hermstad R, Hunskaar S (1995) Female urinary incontinence—consultation behaviour and patient experiences: an epidemiological survey in a Norwegian community. Fam Pract 12:18–21

Shaw C, Tansey R, Jackson C, Hyde C, Allan R (2001) Barriers to help seeking in people with urinary symptoms. Fam Pract 18(1):48–52

Štulhofer A, Hinchliff S, Træen B (2020) Relationship intimacy, sexual distress, and help-seeking for sexual problems among older European couples: a hybrid dyadic approach. Int J Impot Res 32:525–534

Tinetti A, Weir N, Tangyotkajohn U, Jacques A, Thompson J, Briffa K (2018) Help-seeking behaviour for pelvic floor dysfunction in women over 55: drivers and barriers. Int Urogynecol J 29(11):1645–1653

United States Department of Health and Human Services Publications (1992) Urinary incontinence in adults: clinical practice guideline, Washington

Vahdaninia M, Montazeri A, Goshtasebi A (2009) Help-seeking behaviors for female sexual dysfunction: a cross sectional study from Iran. BMC Womens Health 9(1):3

Van der Vaart CH, De Leeuw JRJ, Roovers JPWR, Heintz APM (2002) The effect of urinary incontinence and overactive bladder symptoms on quality of life in young women. BJU Int 90(6):544–549

Batch number: 10091879

Printed by Printforce, the Netherlands